Understanding Biochemical Pathways

A Pattern Recognition Approach

Preliminary Edition

By Carol A. Wilkins
Michigan State University

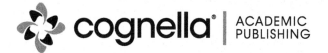

Bassim Hamadeh, CEO and Publisher
Kassie Graves, Director of Acquisitions
Jamie Giganti, Senior Managing Editor
Miguel Macias, Senior Graphic Designer
John Remington, Senior Field Acquisitions Editor
Monika Dziamka, Project Editor
Brian Fahey, Licensing Specialist
Chelsey Schmid, Associate Editor

Cover image copyright © 2013 by iStockphoto LP / isak55.

Printed in the United States of America

ISBN: 978-1-62131-249-9 (pbk) /978-1-62131-250-5 (br)

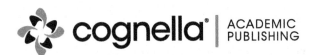

To the Michigan State University College of Human Medicine Advanced Baccalaureate Learning Experience (ABLE) students, Classes of 1998 through 2011

For your "ah-ha" moments that inspired me, and your constant encouragement for me to publish my "recipe" for others to benefit.

To my past and present students in the Michigan State University Colleges of Osteopathic Medicine and Human Medicine

For challenging and inspiring me to continually improve my teaching skills.

Contents

INTRODUCTION i

CHAPTER 1: OXIDATION STATE PATTERNS 1

CHAPTER 2: METABOLISM OVERVIEW AND GLYCOLYSIS 35

CHAPTER 3: MITOCHONDRION OVERVIEW, THE PYRUVATE DEHYDROGENASE COMPLEX, AND THE TCA CYCLE 73

CHAPTER 4: FATTY ACID OXIDATION AND KETONE BODY SYNTHESIS 99

CHAPTER 5: FATTY ACID SYNTHESIS 123

INTRODUCTION

Understanding Biochemical Pathways: A Pattern Recognition Approach is meant to be used **in conjunction with any other complete biochemistry textbook** that is typically required for any level of undergraduate, graduate, or medical school biochemistry course. This is not a "stand-alone" biochemistry textbook. The purpose of this textbook is to provide the reader with a pattern recognition approach to understanding metabolic processes (with the emphasis on human metabolic processes), and it focuses on **specific pathways** of carbohydrate and lipid metabolism that illustrate how to apply this approach. This text presents a "basic recipe" of metabolism to illustrate the general sequence of reactions that are carried out in biochemical pathways to move from one oxidation state of carbon to another. The goal is to give the reader the ability to look at a reaction and determine the type of reaction (based on the differences in reactants and products), the type of enzyme that would catalyze the reaction, and then name the enzyme based on enzyme naming rules. However, this text does <u>not</u> convey or imply the actual enzymatic mechanism by which the reaction is carried out. This text also gives a specific set of questions for the reader to be able to answer regarding any given pathway to assist in understanding the overall "big picture" of the metabolic pathway, and a means for understanding how various metabolic pathways are regulated and integrated.

This text, therefore, presumes the reader is learning (or has learned) certain basic biochemical structures and concepts. These structures include basic structures of amino acids, lipids, nucleotides, and vitamins. The reader should also have knowledge of protein structures, enzyme kinetics, and types of enzyme regulation. The reader should also have an understanding of Gibbs free energy concepts (ΔG), as this plays an important role in understanding how concentration of metabolites can influence the direction in which a reaction proceeds.

This approach is not as simple or easy as one might assume from the standpoint that there is still much to learn about each pathway. This approach will reduce the amount of "rote memorization," which many students feel is the only way to learn metabolic pathways, and achieve better long-term understanding of metabolism. Once one recognizes various patterns in a pathway, key structures, and enzyme naming rules, one can learn the "list of reactions" of a pathway. This is because one has a "picture" of the metabolic pathway that is based on key structures of what has to happen to get from the beginning to the end products of the pathway and the types of reactions and enzymes needed based on the "list".

In using this approach to understanding biochemical pathways, the intent is for the reader to be able to build further upon this knowledge to the extent required by his/her own interest and/or the biochemistry course in which enrolled. Biochemistry is a fascinating and complex subject in which there are many facets that are not fully understood or are being newly discovered. One's understanding of biochemistry will always be advancing. The pattern recognition approach presented in this text will, hopefully, serve as a foundation upon which one can build this additional knowledge.

CHAPTER 1: OXIDATION STATE PATTERNS

Objectives:

1. Define basic organic chemistry terms and apply them to biological reactions. Define the terms: oxidation, reduction, hydration, dehydration, protonate, deprotonate, hydrogen atom, proton, hydride ion, alpha-carbon, beta-carbon, and omega carbon.

2. Recognize the structures of functional groups of carbons and their corresponding prefixes/suffixes used in scientific naming of molecules. Recognize the following functional groups for carbons: alkane, alkene, alcohol [primary (1°), secondary (2°) and tertiary (3°)], aldehyde, ketone, and carboxylic acid; as well as the corresponding suffixes used in naming molecules that will help you to note their presence on biological molecules.

3. Recognize the relationship between corresponding α-amino acids and α-keto acids.

4. Recognize the common reactions used in biological pathways and be able to compare any two of the various functional groups listed in objective #2 to distinguish which of the pair is more oxidized, more reduced, or if they are both at the same oxidation level. Also know the oxidation states of carbons that <u>cannot</u> be further oxidized.

5. Recognize various reaction types, and how the enzymes that carry them out are named: especially regarding dehydrogenases, reductases, kinases, synthases, and synthetases.

6. Diagram the basic reaction patterns needed to oxidize or reduce carbons on a biological molecule.

7. Note that oxidation and reduction reactions are always coupled. Depending on the "direction" of the reaction between two molecules, name the most likely donor or carrier of hydrogen atoms for the reaction (i.e. whether NAD^+/NADH; $NADP^+$/NADPH; or FAD/$FADH_2$ is used).

8. Explain the significance of having a keto group in the α- or β-positions relative to a carboxylic acid.

INTRODUCTION

The first part of this chapter will review some basic concepts and terminology from organic chemistry regarding how to number carbons, recognize key functional groups, and nomenclature tips for naming of molecules. Key organic chemical reactions that are carried out in metabolic pathways will also be reviewed. In the second part of this chapter, a "basic recipe of metabolism" will be presented that will form the basic pattern of reaction sequences that commonly occur in metabolic pathways. An overview of key points in how metabolic pathways work to make energy and the basic rules for naming enzymes are also covered in this chapter.

BASIC CONCEPTS AND TERMINOLOGY

A. Carbon numbering and nomenclature tips

Figure 1.1: Palmitic acid ($C_{16:0}$), a fatty acid

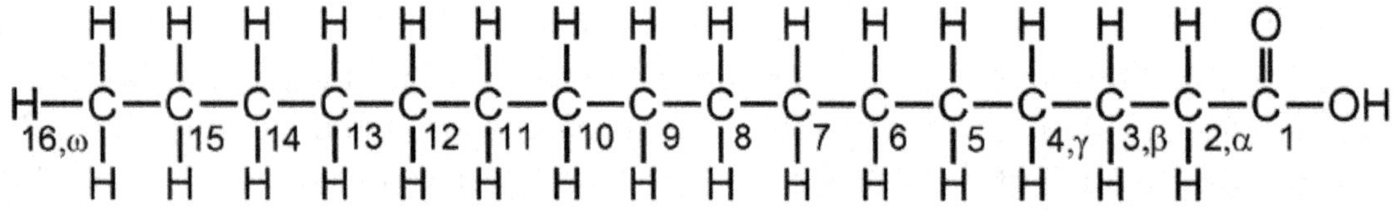

There are two general methods of numbering carbons. For the scientific method of numbering carbons, the carbon with the highest oxidation state, which will be reviewed further in this chapter, is generally designated carbon #1 (or the end carbon nearest the carbon with the highest oxidation state, i.e. the ketoses) and then number the remaining carbons sequentially. For the fatty acid molecule drawn in **Figure 1.1**, the carboxylic acid carbon is the highest oxidation state of carbon in this molecule and thus, is designated carbon #1. The remaining carbons are numbered sequentially to the methyl carbon at the other end, which is carbon #16 for this fatty acid drawn.

Another carbon designation system is often used in reference to biological molecules, which involves designating carbons using Greek letters. This nomenclature is reserved for molecules that have a carboxylic acid. So the carbon of the carboxylic acid is **not** designated with a letter. The carbon **next** to the carboxylic acid carbon is designated "alpha". For the fatty acid drawn above, thus it is carbon #2 that is the "alpha" (α) carbon. Carbon #3 is the beta (β) carbon. This will be important to note when discussing the "beta-oxidation of fatty acids" in which carbon #3 (the beta carbon, is the carbon oxidized). Carbon #4 is the gamma (γ) carbon, and so forth. Using this nomenclature for fatty acids, however, the end methyl carbon of a fatty acid, regardless of its length, is the "omega" (ω) carbon. For the fatty acid shown above, Carbon #16 is the omega (ω) carbon. This terminology is important in understanding the significance of the "omega fatty acids". Omega fatty acids are referring to the relationship of the double bonds in the fatty acid relative to the omega-end of the fatty acid molecule.

For acid groups that are in the protonated state, the molecule is spelled out with "ic acid" as in palmitic acid for the fatty acid drawn in the figure above. Other examples of this nomenclature include acetic acid, pyruvic acid, and lactic acid. When the acid group is in the deprotonated state, COO^-, (the typical state for most acid groups at physiological pH), it is indicated in the molecular name as "ate" (i.e. palmitate, acetate, pyruvate, lactate). Thus the molecular name indicates, already, whether or not it is in the protonated or deprotonated form.

The "yl" ending, which is commonly seen in molecular naming, means that a functional group of a particular molecular is now attached to another molecule. For example, when a fatty acid is attached to another molecule like coenzyme A, the name of the molecule is called "fatty acyl CoA", or often more simply referred to as "acyl CoA". In another example, when three fatty acids are attached to glycerol the name of the new molecule is called a "triacylglycerol". Another important example of this "yl" nomenclature is using acetic acid (or "acetate" for the deprotonated form), which is the shortest fatty acid and is commonly found in biological systems. This fatty acid is two carbons long containing a methyl group attached to the carboxylic acid group. When acetate is attached to coenzyme A, the molecule is called "acetyl CoA", and is a very important intermediate of metabolic pathways.

B. Key reaction definitions

Oxidation, also known as dehydrogenation, is the loss of electrons. For organic reactions, this is loss of hydrogens (notice the whole word "hydrogen" in the name "dehydrogenation"). Hydrogens carry the electrons. There are exceptions to this, but biological systems are not "wires" so they need a carrier of electrons, which are hydrogens. For the oxidation reactions in the most commonly reviewed biochemical pathways (though there are exceptions), these reactions involve the loss of **two** electrons—or loss of **two hydrogens**.

Reduction, also known as hydrogenation, is the gain of electrons. For organic reactions, this is the gain of hydrogens. Again, these reactions generally gain two electrons or hydrogens at a time. Oxidation and reduction reactions are always coupled. Biological systems cannot just let go of electrons and release them, because biological systems are not "metal wires." So if a molecule is oxidized, then another molecule must be reduced (or vice versa). Therefore, these reactions need coenzymes (derived from vitamins) to carry the hydrogens, which include NAD^+, $NADP^+$, FMN, and FAD. These coenzymes are involved in oxidation-reduction reactions because they are carrying the hydrogens to or from an organic molecule. There are many examples which will be reviewed in metabolic reactions. The key point, for now, is to remember that oxidation-reduction reactions are always coupled and are typically referred to as "redox" reactions.

Now contrast oxidation (dehydrogenation) and reduction (hydrogenation) reactions with dehydration and hydration reactions. Dehydration and hydration reactions involve the loss and gain of an entire water molecule, which are **not** redox reactions.

Another set of reactions to differentiate are protonation and deprotonation reactions (see **Figure 1.2**). These reactions involve the gain (protonation) or loss (deprotonation) of protons (H⁺). These reactions are acid-base chemistry, **not** oxidation-reduction reactions, because a proton does not have an electron on it. Therefore proton movement cannot be involved in oxidation-reduction reactions. Thus it is very important to be specific in distinguishing a proton, a hydrogen atom, and a hydride ion and the types of reactions in which they are involved.

Figure 1.2: Protonation/deprotonation reactions

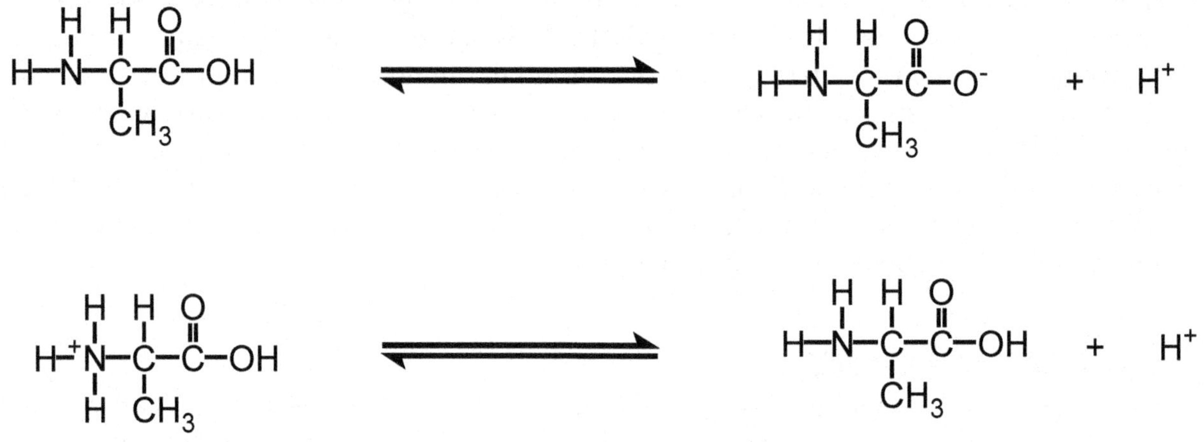

These are acid-base reactions, not oxidation-reduction reactions.

C. Hydrogen terminology

As indicated in **Table 1.1**, a hydrogen atom has one proton and one electron. For organic reactions in most biological systems, hydrogen atoms serve as the carrier of electrons. So to lose electrons from a molecule, the molecule loses hydrogens. If the molecule is gaining electrons, the molecule picks up hydrogens.

Table 1.1: Hydrogen terminology

1.	Hydrogen atom	H = 1 proton and **1** electron
2.	Hydride ion	H^- = 1 proton and **2** electrons
3.	Hydrogen ion (a.k.a. proton)	H^+ = 1 proton and **NO** electrons

A hydride ion is a hydrogen atom carrying **two** electrons (H^-). This is an important point to note for molecules like NAD^+ and $NADP^+$ that have room for only one hydrogen atom.

While the molecule typically loses two hydrogens (i.e. two electrons), NAD⁺ and NADP⁺ then pick up a hydride atom carrying both electrons, and the reaction involves a "leftover proton," as will be explained further in the next section.

A proton, then, is a hydrogen atom that has one proton and **no** electrons. Hence the name "proton", or is also known as a "hydrogen ion." In this text, the term "proton" (H⁺) will be used to prevent confusion with hydride ion. Again, this is why acid-base chemistry (deprotonation-protonation) is different than oxidation-reduction. Acid-base chemistry reactions move protons (not electrons), while oxidation-reduction reactions move electrons (i.e. hydrogen or hydride atoms)

D. Reactions to consider

Vitamins provide the basis for the coenzyme derivatives needed for many reactions. In this chapter, the focus will be on the coenzymes needed for various redox reactions (see **Figure 1.3**). If a molecule is being oxidized, a coenzyme needs to be reduced. If a molecule is being reduced, a coenzyme needs to be oxidized. Throughout metabolic pathways, many examples of these reaction types will be reviewed.

Figure 1.3: Electron transfer of hydrogens, and coenzymes involved in oxidation-reduction reactions.

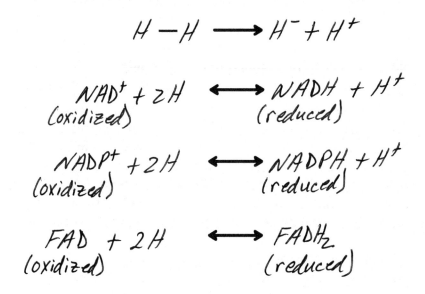

For nicotinamide adenine dinucleotide (NAD⁺), the molecule only has room to accept one hydrogen atom, while the molecule is typically losing two hydrogen atoms. Thus both electrons need to end up on one hydrogen atom, which leaves a leftover proton (NADH + H⁺). This description does not indicate or imply anything about the actual enzyme mechanisms by which these reactions occur. Rather the reader should note the establishment of the "pattern" of noting how many hydrogens are lost or gained from an organic molecule, as well as the type of electron carrier accepted or lost by the coenzyme (i.e. either two actual hydrogen atoms, or a hydride ion plus a leftover proton). Nicotinamide adenine dinucleotide phosphate ($NADP^+$) carries out the same reaction as NAD^+, because $NADP^+$ is the same molecule except it has a phosphate "tag" as part of its structure.

Another reason to note that electrons can be stripped from a hydrogen atom to produce a proton is to ultimately lead into the concept of proton "pumping" in the electron transport chain. The basic concept of the electron transport chain (ETC) is the same, move the electron off of a hydrogen atom because some of the coenzymes in the electron transport chain only accept electrons (because they do contain metal atoms), resulting in production of a proton—which ultimately produces the proton gradient. The vitamin riboflavin is converted into two coenzyme derivatives: flavin adenine dinucleotide (FAD) and flavin mononucleotide (FMN). Both, which have the same functional part of the molecule, have room for both hydrogen atoms that are lost from a molecule. So FAD and FMN get reduced to $FADH_2$ and $FMNH_2$, respectively.

NADH and $FADH_2$ are commonly referred to as "reducing power" because NADH and $FADH_2$ are the carriers of hydrogens (electrons) to the electron transport chain (ETC). Therefore, NADH and $FADH_2$ are "reducing power" because they are carrying electrons that can be given to another molecule to "reduce it" in the ETC, which is the pathway that produces the majority of ATP from the catabolism of biological molecules. NADPH, on the other hand, is the form of reducing power used for synthetic reactions, overall. There are always exceptions to these rules, but NADPH is not used as an electron donor to the ETC.

E. Primary, secondary, and tertiary designations of alcohols

Another set of basic chemistry terminology to review is the designation of primary, secondary, tertiary alcohols (see **Figure 1.4**). In this case, the designation is based on the carbon with the hydroxy group (-OH) on it. If this carbon is attached to only one other carbon, it is a primary alcohol. If the hydroxy carbon is attached to two other carbons, it is a secondary alcohol. If the hydroxy carbon is attached to three other carbons, it is a tertiary alcohol. The key to note here is that tertiary alcohols CANNOT be further oxidized. For example in the tricarboxylic acid (TCA) cycle, the reason why citrate must be isomerized to isocitrate is because citrate contains a tertiary alcohol.

Figure 1.4: Primary, secondary and tertiary alcohols

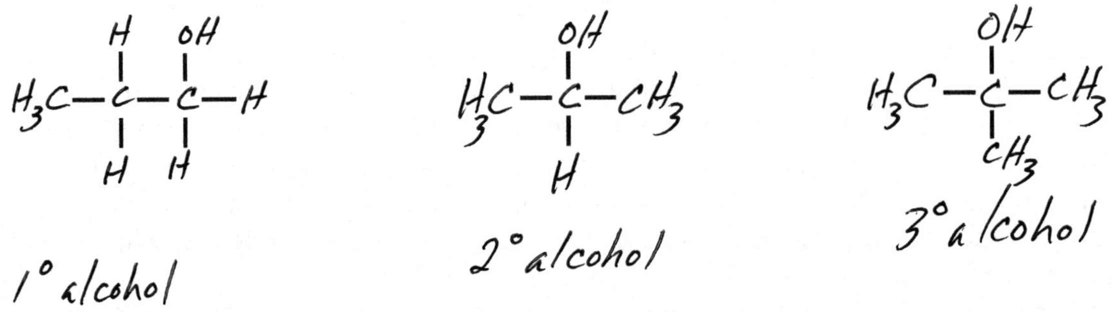

F. Relationship between α-amino acids and α-keto acids

Recall the alpha (α) carbon is the carbon next to a carboxylic acid. In **Figure 1.5** the α-keto acids are drawn on the left. These molecules must have a keto-group next to a carboxylic acid. Ketones must be "in the middle" of a molecule where carbonyl carbon (C double bond O) is attached to two other carbons (recall carbons can only make 4 bonds).

Figure 1.5: Relationship between α-keto acids and α-amino acids

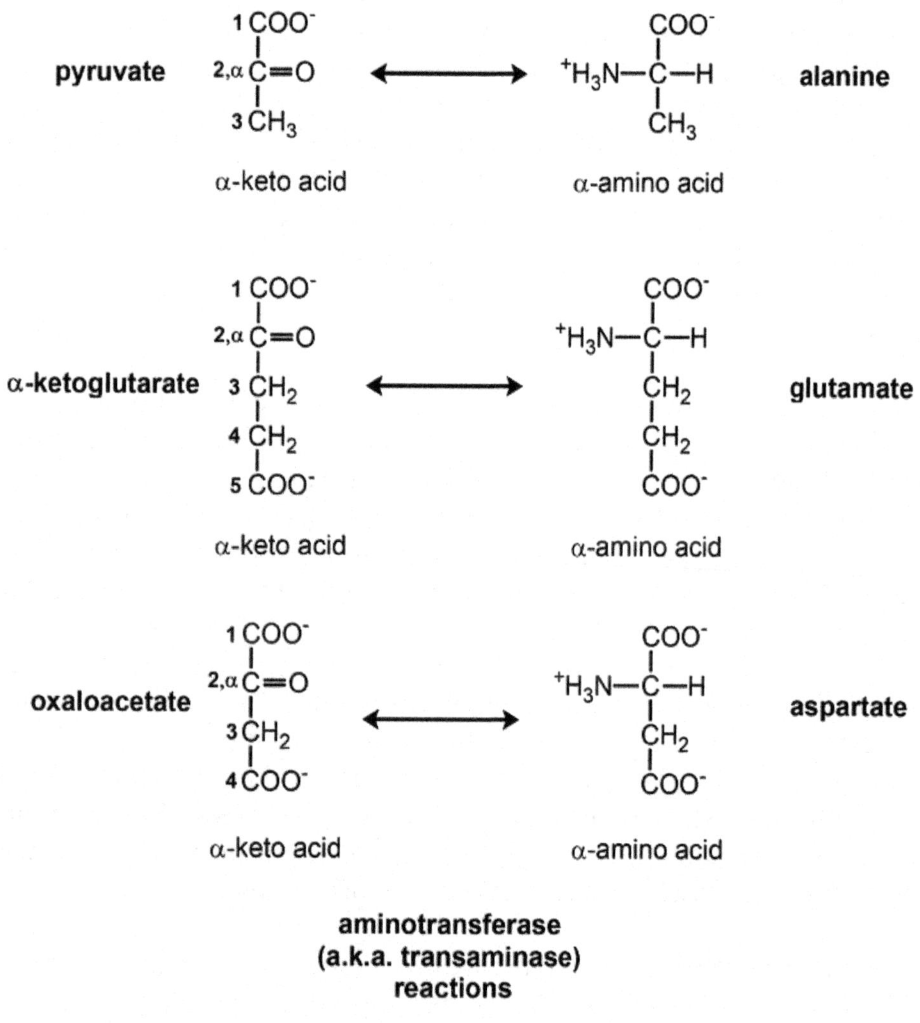

aminotransferase
(a.k.a. transaminase)
reactions

For the top left molecule of **Figure 1.5** is pyruvate, an α-keto acid. While its name does not tell indicate much about its structure (other than the fact that it has a carboxyl group that is in the deprotonated state), pyruvate is such a key molecule in metabolism that pyruvate is absolutely one of the key structures the reader should know (i.e. be able to draw it, as well as recognize it).

Now "replace" the α-keto groups for the molecules on the left of **Figure 1.5** with an amino group and a hydrogen atom, which results in the molecules drawn on the right. These are now amino acids, which have attached to the α-carbon: a carboxylic acid, an amino group, a hydrogen, and an R group. The amino acid drawn at the top right is alanine. So this is the simplest way to convert amino acids to something else. Simply "remove" the amino group off to produce the corresponding α-keto acid or create a new amino acid by putting an amino group on an α-keto acid. Thus, this is the relationship between corresponding α-keto acids and α-amino acids. Again, this description is not intended to imply anything about the enzyme mechanism by which this done, only noting the structural pattern between α-keto acids and α-amino acids. The reaction that accomplishes this interchange is called transamination, which is carried out by enzymes called aminotransferases (or in some older texts, the enzymes are called transaminases).

Now let us look at a couple of other corresponding α-keto acids and α-amino acids. For another nomenclature hint: anytime the prefix "glut" is in a molecular name—think 5 carbons. For the middle left molecule drawn in **Figure 1.5**, the carbons are numbered 1 through 5 (as shown), with a keto-group on carbon #2 (the α-carbon) producing an α-keto acid, termed α-keto<u>glut</u>arate. If the α-keto group is replaced with an amino group and a hydrogen, the corresponding α-amino acid—<u>glut</u>amate—is produced (shown in **Figure 1.5**).

The bottom set of molecules drawn in **Figure 1.5** is the α-keto acid, oxaloacetate, and its corresponding α-amino acid, aspartate. Again, the exchange of a keto functionality for an amino group and hydrogen atom differentiates the two molecules. Both α-ketoglutarate and oxaloacetate are TCA cycle intermediates. Thus, knowing the relationships between α-amino acids and α-keto acids will provide "straightforward" connections to amino acid synthesis and amino acid breakdown pathways.

If the reader is not required to draw structures on assignments or examinations, rather he/she must be able to "recognize" them; learning structural patterns will help the reader differentiate structures without necessarily being able to draw entire molecules (and requires less rote memorization of structures). For instance, glutamate and aspartate are the two amino acids which have carboxylic acid functionalities as part of their R groups. Remembering that "glut" means five carbons, one needs to recognize the basic structure of an amino acid to determine the R group portion. If the R group ends in a carboxylic acid functional group and has a total of five carbons (including the α-carboxylic acid group carbon), the amino acid must be glutamate. If it ends in a carboxylic acid functional group, but is not five carbons, then it must be the "other one"—aspartate (which has four carbons total).

Whether or not the reader is or is not required to draw structures, wherever possible let the name of the molecule indicate the actual structure of the molecule. First learn key structures, which will be indicated throughout this text. Then by learning patterns of structures, as well as how molecules are named, recognition or drawing of other "derivatives" of those key structures will become more straightforward. For example, if one can draw glutamate as its five carbon structure, simply note that aspartate is basically "missing" one CH_2 group (rather than memorize these two entire structures as separate entities).

OXIDATION STATES FLOW CHART ("BASIC RECIPE OF METABOLISM")

The following section will cover the oxidation states flow chart, or what I have termed the "basic recipe of metabolism." IMPORTANT NOTE: In the discussion of the reactions of this oxidation states flow chart, _nowhere_ are the actual enzymatic mechanisms being implied or described. This basic recipe of metabolism simply lays out the pattern of organic reactions that are carried out in humans (and many other organisms), the typical coenzymes needed, and the relationships of the types of reactions used by the body to get carbons to the various oxidation states.

The reader must first be able to recognize the difference between the various functional groups: an alkane, an alkene, an alcohol, a keto group, an aldehyde, a carboxylic acid group. These are all various oxidation states of carbon, and are indicated in **Figure 1.6**. **Figure 1.6** also indicates the common suffixes used in naming conventions to identify various functional groups as components of molecules. This figure indicates the oxidation states of the various functional groups in relation to one another, which is organized from fully reduced to fully oxidized molecules. Functionalities at the same oxidation level are indicated. Full oxidation of a 3 carbon alkane to 3 molecules of CO_2 would indicate complete oxidation of the all the carbons. Breathing off of these 3 molecules of CO_2 would mean that the body has completely removed this molecule from the body.

Many molecules have more than one functional group, or even more than one of the same functional group. So when one is trying to determine what type of reaction is happening to go from one molecule to the next—focus on what is **_different_** between the molecules. If the starting and ending molecules have same number of each atom, rearranged, they have been isomerized. If the starting molecule does not have a phosphate group and the product does, the molecule has been phosphorylated. If the phosphate group has been removed, it is a dephosphorylation reaction. If the only difference between the starting and ending molecules is the number of hydrogens, it is an oxidation-reduction reaction. The metabolic pathways contain many examples of these types of reactions, and will be reviewed in the context of the oxidation states flow chart ("the basic recipe of metabolism"), which is covered in the next section.

Figure 1.6: Nomenclature of oxidation states and suffixes

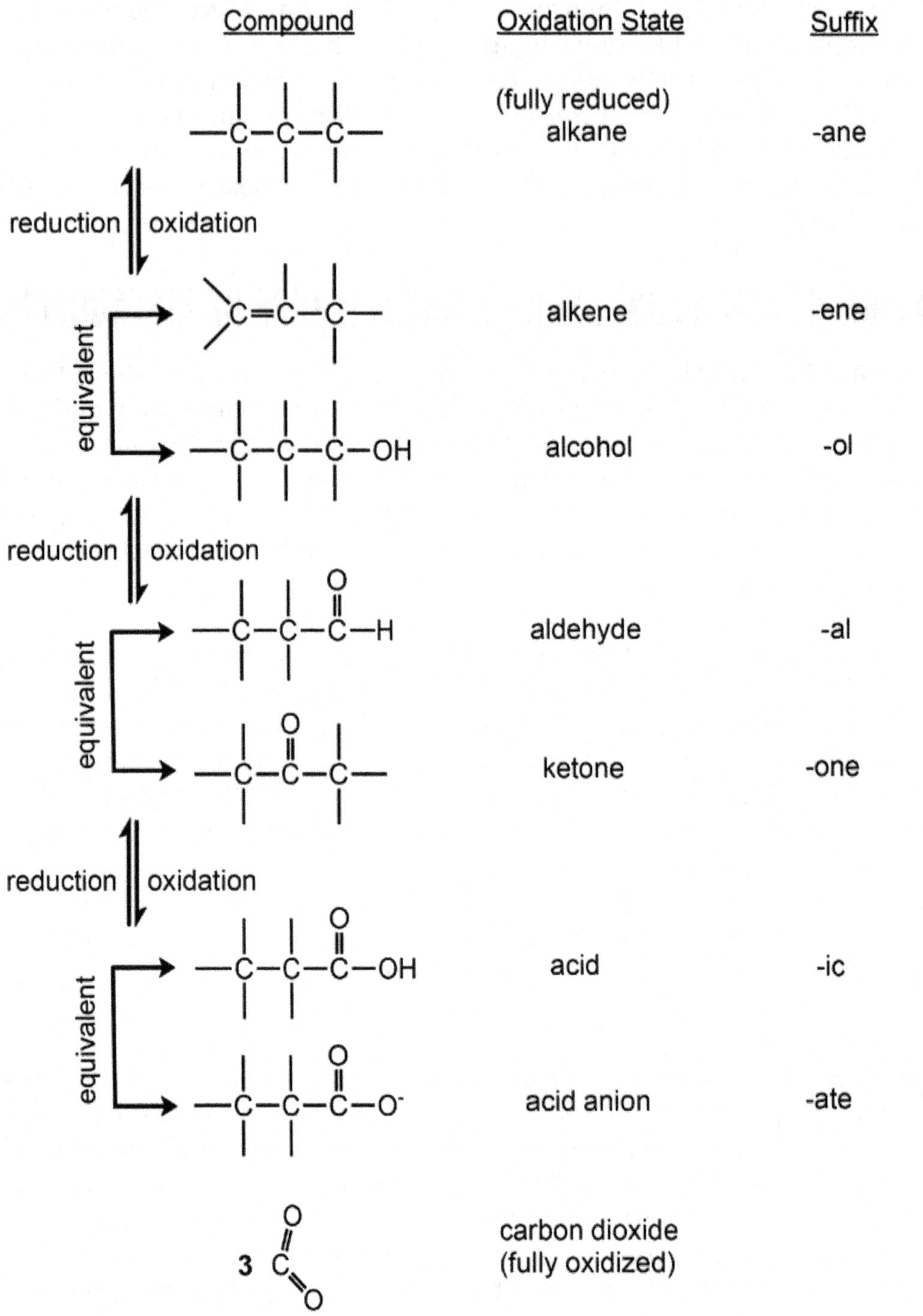

Compound	Oxidation State	Suffix
—C—C—C—	(fully reduced) alkane	-ane
C=C—C—	alkene	-ene
—C—C—C—OH	alcohol	-ol
—C—C—C—H (O)	aldehyde	-al
—C—C—C— (O)	ketone	-one
—C—C—C—OH (O)	acid	-ic
—C—C—C—O⁻ (O)	acid anion	-ate
3 C (O, O)	carbon dioxide (fully oxidized)	

Other suffixes:
(1) -ase   enzyme
(2) -ose   sugar
(3) -yl   a functional group in a bond with another functional group

Figure 1.7, on the next page, is the key figure termed the "Oxidation States Flow Chart". This flow chart of reactions is what I often refer to as "the basic recipe of metabolism." The oxidation states flow chart, as stated, does not refer to actual mechanisms. Rather the flow chart indicates the set of commonly repeated reactions that occur, often in sequence, in numerous metabolic pathways. These reactions are most often seen in the pathways of catabolism or synthesis of monosaccharides, fatty acids, and amino acids. In the following chapters of this text, examples of how to recognize these reactions individually and/or in sequence will be demonstrated using common metabolic pathways covered in biochemistry. This will, hopefully, provide the reader with a basic foundation upon which to further learn additional pathways, and to build subsequent knowledge regarding the complexity and integration biochemical pathways.

The orientation of the functional groups drawn in the oxidation flow chart is organized with the most reduced molecule at the top of the **Figure 1.7**. The most oxidized molecule is at the bottom of the figure. As one moves down the page, the molecules are becoming more oxidized relative to one another. As one moves up the page, the molecules are becoming more reduced. Molecules drawn at the same level horizontally across the page are at equivalent oxidation states (i.e. the types of reactions needed to convert them are hydrations/dehydrations or isomerizations, **not** redox reactions).

At the top of the oxidation states flow chart (**Figure 1.7**) is drawn an alkane, which is the most reduced state of carbon. An alkane is basically a carbon making 4 single bonds (the maximum it can make) to either carbons or hydrogens only. Thus, the three carbons in the alkane drawn are all at the most reduced oxidation state. The ultimate goal in catabolic biological pathways is to oxidize carbons to carboxylic acids, which can be clipped off and transported in the blood back to the lungs to be exhaled from the body, and produce "reducing power" in the form of NADH and $FADH_2$.

Figure 1.7: Oxidation States Flow Chart (the "Basic Recipe" of Metabolism)

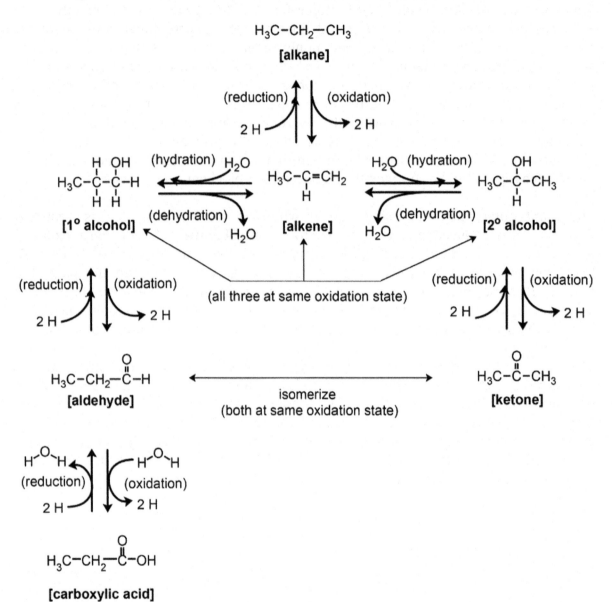

The reactions in the oxidation states flow chart will now be separated out to review them individually or in smaller sets. In each reaction covered, the substrates and products will be drawn to match the oxidation states flow chart. The first reaction is the oxidation of the alkane to the alkene, shown in **Figure 1.8**.

Figure 1.8: The oxidation of an alkane to alkene (and reverse reaction).

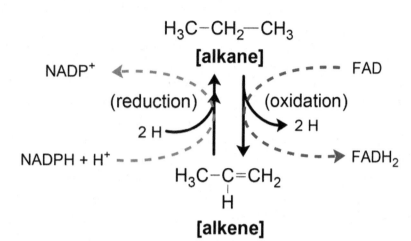

[alkene]

The alkane drawn has three carbons and eight hydrogens. The alkane is converted to an alkene, which has a double bond between two carbon atoms (general formula: $R_2C=CR_2$). The alkene now has three carbons, but only 6 hydrogens. In this reaction, the alkane has lost two hydrogens to become an alkene. Therefore this is an oxidation-reduction reaction. So the alkene is now *oxidized* relative to the alkane. However, as previously mentioned, molecules in biological systems do not just "lose hydrogens" (i.e. electrons)—the hydrogens must go somewhere. The first general rule for coenzyme use in redox reaction: Any time an alkane is oxidized to an alkene, FAD is used as the coenzyme. FAD is reduced to $FADH_2$. Recall that oxidation and reduction reactions are always coupled. Note that the indication of "oxidization" next to the down arrow of the reaction (**Figure 1.8**) is relative to what is happening to the organic molecule (i.e. the alkane to alkene comparison). Again, a coenzyme must always be used to accept the hydrogens (i.e. be reduced). This chart is **not** implying the actual enzymatic mechanism that takes place for the transfer of the hydrogens from the alkane to FAD. Just note the pattern, and that the coenzyme of the enzymes that carry out the oxidation of alkanes to alkenes is FAD, which gets reduced to $FADH_2$. FAD is also used as a coenzyme for other types of reactions in other enzymes (i.e. the pyruvate dehydrogenase complex, and the α-ketoglutarate dehydrogenase complex).

Since the other oxidation states of carbon have oxygens, oxygens will need to be added to the molecule to get the carbons to these other oxidation states. Water molecules will be used to add these oxygens. One must further note that biochemical pathways cannot go directly from an alkane to an alcohol. The alkane must be oxidized to the alkene, first. Once the alkene is produced, then the alcohol functionality can be formed.

Now consider the reactions that convert the alkene to an alcohol, shown below in **Figure 1.9**. An alcohol is a molecule with a hydroxy group (-OH). Thus, to convert the alkene to an alcohol requires the addition of an entire molecule of water. In the hydration reactions drawn in **Figure 1.9**, an entire water molecule is added across the double bond, with the placement of an –OH on one carbon, and the remaining hydrogen on the other carbon. Depending on where the –OH group is placed depends on whether a primary alcohol or secondary alcohol is produced, which was defined previously. If the hydroxy group is placed on the end carbon, as drawn to the left in **Figure 1.9**, a primary (1º) alcohol is produced. If the hydroxy group is placed on the middle carbon, as drawn to the right in **Figure 1.9**, a secondary (2º) alcohol is produced. Tertiary (3º) alcohols can also be formed (not shown), but tertiary alcohols cannot be further oxidized as previously mentioned. Note that the alcohols and alkene are drawn at the same level horizontally, meaning they are all at the same oxidation state.

Figure 1.9: The interconversion of alkenes and alcohols.

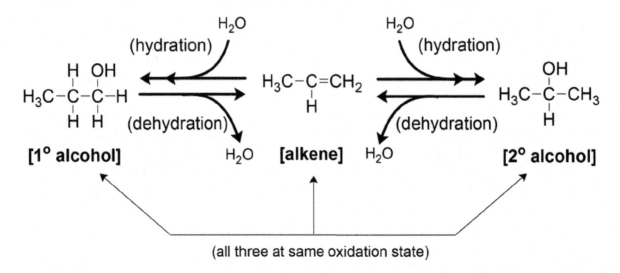

Now consider the secondary alcohol, which can be further oxidized. In the reaction drawn in **Figure 1.10**, simply count the hydrogens. Notice that two hydrogens from the secondary alcohol are lost (one from the hydroxy group and one from the center carbon—again, not mechanistically correct), forming a carbonyl group (a.k.a. a keto-group, or ketone). A C=O is a carbonyl carbon. There are many functional groups that have a carbonyl group (i.e. aldehydes and carboxylic acids), but a keto-group is "*just*" a carbonyl group (C=O) with the carbon bound to 2 other carbons.

Since the only difference between the secondary alcohol and the ketone drawn in **Figure 1.10** is the loss of two hydrogens, this is an oxidation reaction. These two hydrogens must be added to a coenzyme. In this case the coenzyme is NAD^+ (oxidized form), which is reduced to $NADH + H^+$. Remember there is always a leftover proton, as NAD^+ picks up a hydride ion carrying both electrons. In fact NAD^+ is the coenzyme for all of the remaining oxidation reactions going "down" the flow chart. FAD is only used for the alkane to alkene reaction.

Figure 1.10: The oxidation of a secondary alcohol to a ketone (and the reverse reaction).

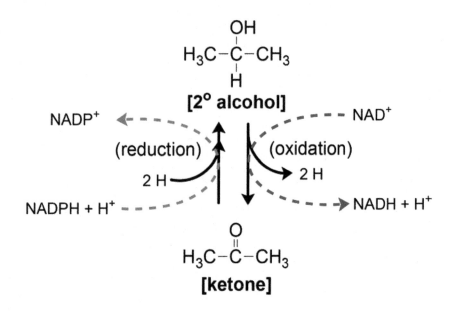

The ketone shown in this **Figure 1.10** reaction is acetone, which is the simplest ketone. Acetone is a key molecule to know (both its name and its molecular structure) because it is the basis of naming of other structures, as well as one of the ketone bodies. Ketones **cannot** be further oxidized. Thus, there are two functionalities to note that cannot be further oxidized, ketones and tertiary (3°) alcohols. Fructose, a ketose sugar, is considered a reducing sugar. A reducing sugar is a sugar that can be oxidized, and thus reduce another molecule in the process. Fructose, in an alkaline solution, is in equilibrium with an aldehyde through an enediol intermediate. Thus, fructose still essentially "follows the rule" that a ketone needs to be isomerized to an aldehyde before becoming oxidized to a carboxylic acid.

The aldehyde drawn on the left of the oxidation states chart (**Figure 1.7**) can be produced in two ways. First, consider the reaction of the primary alcohol drawn in **Figure 1.11**. Again, compare the structure of the primary alcohol and the aldehyde drawn. Aldehyde functional groups must be on an end carbon (by definition of the molecular structure, -CH=O). Count the number of hydrogens on the primary alcohol and on the aldehyde and note that two hydrogens have been removed, one from the hydroxy group and one from that end carbon itself (again, not implying the actual mechanism). Those two hydrogens must go somewhere—i.e. onto a coenzyme. As mentioned previously, NAD$^+$ will be the coenzyme, which gets reduced to NADH + H$^+$. To go from a primary alcohol to an aldehyde is an oxidation reaction, indicating that the aldehyde is more oxidized than the alcohol.

Figure 1.11: The oxidation of a primary alcohol to an aldehyde (and the reverse reaction).

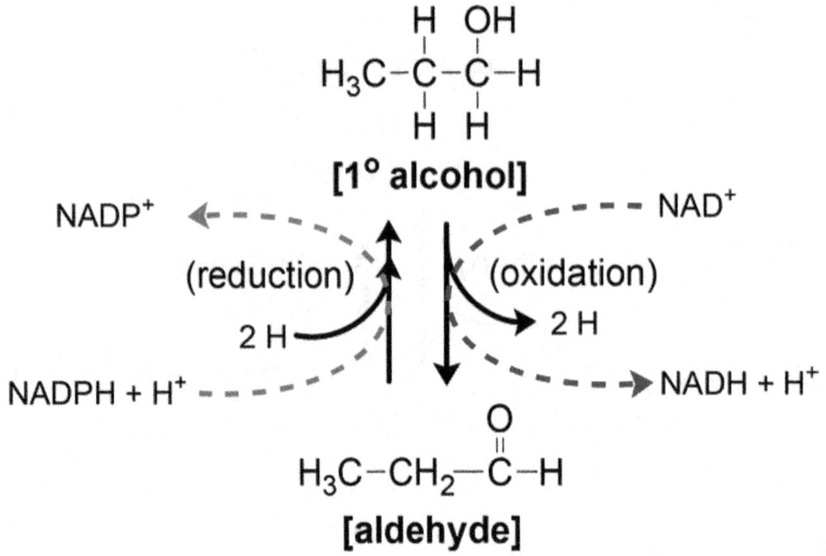

The same aldehyde on the flow chart (**Figure 1.7**) can be produced by another reaction. In this case, start with the ketone drawn (acetone) in the reaction shown in **Figure 1.12**. The three-carbon aldehyde and the three-carbon ketone have the same number of carbons, hydrogens, and oxygens. Therefore, these two molecules can be interchanged by isomerization reactions. There are many enzymes that can simply isomerize a ketone functionality to an aldehyde functionality (and vice versa). For example, fructose (a ketose sugar) and glucose (an aldose, or aldehyde, sugar) are both $C_6H_{12}O_6$ molecules. They have the same number of carbons, hydrogens, and oxygens, but they are arranged differently. Thus fructose and glucose are isomers of one another. It is simply a "switch" of the carbon functionalities on carbons 1 and 2 of these molecules. Thus aldehydes and ketones, with all component atoms being equal in number, are at the same oxidation level.

Figure 1.12: The interconversion of aldehydes and ketones.

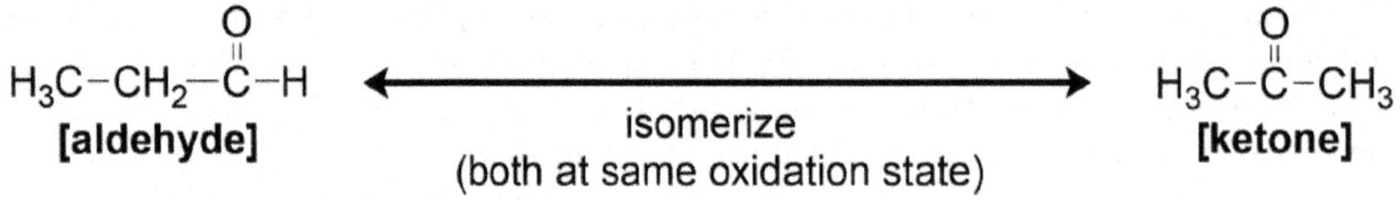

The last oxidation reaction will get a carbon to the highest oxidation state of carbon—the carboxylic acid group (COOH, or COO-). Getting carbons oxidized to carboxylic acids is the goal of catabolic pathways. The carboxylic acid group can be clipped off as carbon dioxide (CO_2), under certain conditions, and is the primary way which carbon is excreted by breathing it out from the lungs. The carboxylic acid group is the most oxidized state of carbon that is still attached to a molecule because CO_2, by itself, is truly the most oxidized state of carbon.

For the aldehyde to carboxylic acid reaction shown in **Figure 1.13**, a molecule of water is required because another oxygen is needed. However, this is *not* a hydration reaction because only "part" of the water molecule is added. The structure of the carboxylic acid group, compared to the aldehyde group, looks like an –OH group has "replaced" the hydrogen of the aldehyde. Thus, count the number of hydrogens from both the aldehyde AND the water molecule and compare to the number of hydrogens on the molecule with the carboxylic acid. There are six hydrogens on the molecule with the carboxylic acid. There are eight hydrogens between the molecule with the aldehyde and the water molecule. Thus, there is a loss of two hydrogens—just from two DIFFERENT molecules—one from the aldehyde group and the other from the water molecule. Again, the hydrogens have to go somewhere, to the coenzyme of choice: NAD^+. NAD^+ gets reduced to $NADH + H^+$. Therefore the conversion of an aldehyde to a carboxylic acid is an oxidation reaction, coupled with the reduction of a coenzyme.

Figure 1.13: The oxidation of an aldehyde to a carboxylic acid (and the reverse reaction).

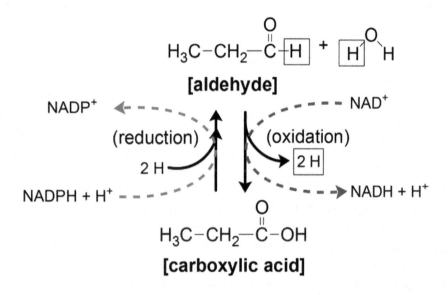

Before discussing what happens with the carboxylic acid group that has been formed on the molecule, consider now the reverse reactions to go "up" the oxidation states flow chart. Biochemical pathways can go "back" from carboxylic acids and the other functionalities, to get back to any of the other oxidation states, including all the way back to an alkane. Typically this occurs in synthetic pathways. Most synthetic pathways are *reductive* pathways to get carbons to a more reduced state (i.e. fatty acid synthesis, which requires the reduction of keto groups back to alkanes). When going "up" the oxidation chart, a coenzyme must donate the hydrogens to the molecule to reduce it. The coenzyme of choice: NADPH (reduced form). Recall that $NADP^+$/NADPH is the same as NAD^+/NADH, with the addition of a phosphate "tag." Think of the phosphate "tag" as a means to indicate that this molecule is to be used for synthetic reactions (going up). NADPH is **not** a donor of hydrogens to the electron transport chain. So everywhere a reduction is shown on the reverse reactions in the previous reaction **Figures 1.8, 1.10, 1.11 and 1.13**, NADPH (reduced form) + H^+ is oxidized to $NADP^+$ (as indicated in the reactions going "up"). This <u>includes</u> reducing alkenes back to alkanes (i.e. no new coenzyme is needed for this last reduction). The reactions to go from the alcohols to the alkene are dehydration reactions (not redox reactions), which is the loss of water.

Now that all of the reactions of the oxidation states flow chart have been covered, individually, review the entire sequence of reactions in **Figure 1.7**. Note, in particular, how the reactions are related to one another going "down" the oxidation states flow chart (oxidizing), as well as going "up" the chart (reducing). Also note the relationship of the functional groups to one another, and the coenzymes needed for the reactions. These concepts will be related to the biochemical pathways covered in the remaining chapters of this text to provide the reader with a means to understanding the reactions that take place in a particular pathway and why the reactions proceed in a particular order. These are the "patterns of biochemical pathways".

There is also a defined protocol for naming the enzymes of the biochemical pathways. While the enzyme naming rules will make more sense as when covering the actual enzymes involved in metabolic pathways, a general overview of oxidation-reduction (redox) reaction enzyme naming is presented here. Generally speaking, the easiest way to remember how to name redox enzymes is as follows:

1. Enzymes that use $NADP^+$/NADPH (regardless of which direction the reaction goes, because many redox reactions are reversible)—are called **reductases** and are *named for the more oxidized molecule* because that is the molecule that is being reduced.

2. Enzymes that use FAD/$FADH_2$ or NAD^+/NADH (again, regardless of which direction the reaction is being carried out) are called **dehydrogenases** (recall oxidation is also called dehydrogenation—loss of hydrogens). Dehydrogenases are *named for the more reduced molecule* because that is the molecule that is being oxidized (dehydrogenated) by the enzyme based on its name.

These are the general rules of the oxidation states flow chart and the redox enzyme naming conventions. There will be some exceptions, but if the reader knows the rules—one just needs to remember the few exceptions (i.e. if "it" was not learned as an exception, "it" must follow the rule).

DECARBOXYLATIONS AND KEY STRATEGIES FOR MAKING ENERGY

Now consider what happens to the carboxylic acid group that has been formed from all the oxidation steps covered to get from the alkane to the carboxylic acid. Once that carboxylic acid formed, the goal is to clip it off and then transport it through the blood back to the lungs to be breathed off as CO_2. One does not keep every molecule of carbon, oxygen, hydrogen, etc. that is obtained from nutrients in a lifetime. Carbon dioxide (CO_2) is one of the major mechanisms of excreting carbons and oxygens in animals (and other organisms). The problem is that carboxyl acid groups are stable. They are not good leaving groups. A basic rule of organic chemistry—functional groups cannot just "be removed" from a molecule, unless they are good leaving groups. To get rid of the carboxylic group as a good leaving group, another reaction will have to be carried out on the molecule to make it a good leaving group.

A. Decarboxylation of carboxylic acid groups (R-COOH ➔ RH + CO$_2$)

To remove a carboxylic acid group from a molecule (i.e. decarboxylation reaction) in biological pathways, an alpha (α) or beta (β) keto acid is produced. In **Figure 1.14** the first molecule drawn is a very short (four-carbon) fatty acid.

Figure 1.14: Stability of carboxylic acid groups on a fatty acid

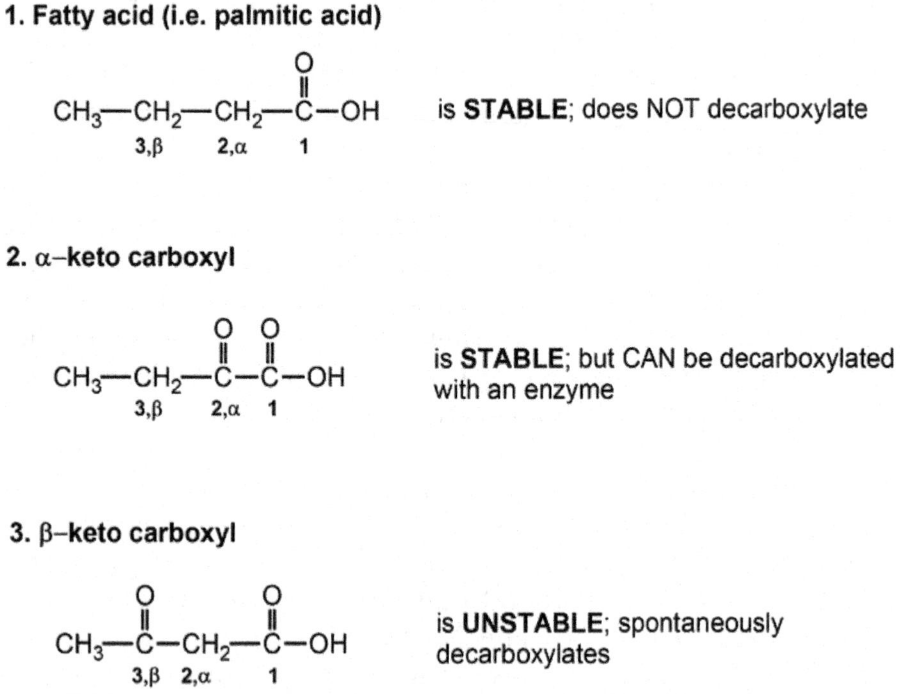

1. Fatty acid (i.e. palmitic acid)

is **STABLE**; does NOT decarboxylate

2. α–keto carboxyl

is **STABLE**; but CAN be decarboxylated with an enzyme

3. β–keto carboxyl

is **UNSTABLE**; spontaneously decarboxylates

A fatty acid molecule is very stable, and it does not spontaneously decarboxylate. To make the carboxylic acid group a good leaving group, a keto group is put nearby. The keto group can be put on either the α-carbon (recall that is carbon #2 using scientific numbering) or the β-carbon (carbon #3). If the keto group is placed on the α-carbon (shown in **Figure 1.14**), the carboxylic acid group is still stable, but can be decarboxylated with an enzyme complex. The basic point is that the decarboxylation of α-keto acids is very "difficult" and requires a large enzyme complex (i.e. the pyruvate dehydrogenase complex and the α-ketoglutarate dehydrogenase complex). While α-keto acids can be decarboxylated, a better option—if possible—is to put the keto group on the β-carbon (shown in **Figure 1.14**). Beta-keto acids are unstable and will spontaneously decarboxylate. Note that "spontaneous" does not mean "instantaneous." Spontaneous does not indicate anything about the reaction rate. The decarboxylation of β-keto acids still generally requires an enzyme to move the reaction along in most biological pathways. For β-keto acids, the carboxylic acid is now a good leaving group, and can "leave" the molecule without the need of an enzyme. One example is the ketone body, acetone, which is formed from the spontaneous decarboxylation of the ketone body, acetoacetate (a β-keto acid). Ketone bodies are an important water-soluble fuel source for the body derived from the catabolism of fatty acids. Acetone, though, can only be excreted. It cannot be used as a fuel source.

B. Key strategies for making energy (ATP)

GOAL: Make NADH, FADH₂, which is used by the ETC to make ATP

This overall scheme for making energy is a *very* simplistic view, and is based on patterns—not mechanisms. The goal of catabolic processes is to oxidize the carbons organic molecules by removing hydrogens (dehydrogenation). Remember FAD as the coenzyme for the oxidation of alkanes to alkenes because FAD can accept two hydrogens from the two different carbons of the alkane to be reduced to $FADH_2$. (Note, the actual reason is the reducing power of alkanes is not sufficient to reduce NAD^+ to NADH). For the oxidation of alcohols and aldehydes, the coenzyme used is NAD^+ because the reactions remove hydrogen(s) from one carbon, and NAD^+ can only accept one hydrogen atom (as a hydride ion carrying both electrons). *Also note*: the oxidation of aldehydes generally yields a high energy bond "S—P" which can be used for *substrate level phosphorylation* to yield ATP (or an energy equivalent).

As noted, the carboxylic acid is the most oxidized state of carbon on a molecule. Notice on the oxidation chart, every time a molecule was oxidized—a coenzyme was reduced. Again, oxidation (going down the page) is what catabolic pathways accomplish. The more oxidations needed to get a carbon to the carboxylic acid functionality, the more $FADH_2$ and NADH produced. $FADH_2$ and NADH are the substrates for the electron transport chain (ETC), which is the major producer of ATP for a cell. The more $FADH_2$ and NADH produced by a catabolic pathway means that more ATP can be made by the ETC. This is the goal of catabolism: to make reducing power ($FADH_2$ and NADH) produced by oxidation reactions that in turn can by used by the ETC to make ATP. In addition, the products of the catabolic pathways are waste products that can be excreted (i.e. CO_2, H_2O, and NH_4^+ for nitrogen-containing molecules). Catabolic processes, then, produce lots of CO_2, acids and protons (H^+) that affect the pH of blood.

The more reduced the molecule, the more oxidations that have to be done to get each carbon up to a carboxylic acid. Thus the more reduced molecules ultimately provide more $FADH_2$ and NADH to the ETC for ATP production. Hence fatty acids will ultimately produce more ATP per molecule than a molecule of glucose (sugar). The carbons on sugars like glucose (6 carbons) are alcohols or aldehydes and do not require as many oxidations to get rid of a glucose. For a fatty acid like palmitate (a C_{16} fatty acid), there are 15 carbons at the level of an alkane and one carbon is a carboxylic acid. Therefore, many more oxidations are required to get rid of palmitate. Hopefully, after covering carbohydrate versus fatty acid catabolism in the subsequent chapter of this book, one will truly understand why a fatty acid molecule will ultimately yield more ATP than a molecule of glucose.

NAMING OF ENZYMES

The general classifications and rules for naming enzymes are outlined below. These rules will be covered in more detail using the actual enzyme names of the metabolic pathways covered in this text.

I. Six Functional Classification Groups of Enzymes
  A. Oxido-reductases
  1. Catalyze oxidation-reduction reactions (a.k.a. redox reactions)
  2. *Oxidation*—**removal of electrons (molecule becomes more +)**
  3. *Reduction*—**addition of electrons (molecule becomes more -)**
  4. NOTE: (for the readers who have difficulty seeing an "addition" of something as a "reduction") electrons are **negatively** charged, so the "addition" of electrons to a molecule makes the charge **more negative** (or less positive)—i.e. "**reduced**"
  5. Know "oxidation states flow chart"
  6. These enzymes are called **dehydrogenases** = removal of hydrogens. (Hydrogen is the carrier of the electrons—usually; an exception—the ETC complexes.)
  7. The enzymes require a **coenzyme**, which acts as a donor or acceptor of the electrons (carried by hydrogens; again except ETC complexes—many of the complexes use various metal ions as coenzymes for electron movement).

  B. Transferases
  1. Transfers a functional group from one compound to another compound.
  2. Example: a **kinase** = an enzyme that transfers phosphate (PO_4) groups.

  C. Hydrolases
  1. Breaks bonds by the addition of H_2O.
  2. Dehydrolases—remove H_2O from a compound(s)

  D. Lyases
  1. Breaks bonds (without the addition of H_2O)

2. Forms double bonds (<u>note</u>—double bonds also can be formed by oxidation-reduction reactions)

E. Isomerases
1. Catalyzes the formation of isomers of a compound (configurational change)
2. ***Isomers*** = same number of atoms and bonds, but in a different configuration.

F. Ligases
1. Makes bonds using energy (ATP)

G. **NOTE:**
1. Transferases and Ligases are two classes of enzymes that can make <u>big</u> molecules (i.e. make bonds).
2. Hydrolases and Lyases are two classes of enzymes that break bonds.

II. Rules for Naming Enzymes
A. Suffix for all enzymes is <u>**-ase**</u>.

B. Anabolic (Synthetic) Reactions:
  1. Name product
  2. Followed by either (a) Synthase—no energy required (classified—<u>transferase</u>)
  3. <u>OR</u> (b) Synthetase—energy required (classified—<u>ligase</u>)

C. Catabolic (Breakdown) Reactions:
  1. Name reactant(s)
  2. Followed by the type of reaction being carried out.

D. Oxido-reductase enzymes (a.k.a. redox enzymes)
  1. For ***CATABOLIC*** pathways
     a. Name the **reduced** molecule
     b. Followed by <u>dehydrogenase</u>
     c. **UNLESS** molecular oxygen is used directly in which you then follow it by <u>oxidase</u>
     d. Note: When multiple reactions are carried out by an enzyme, if any one of the reactions is redox, then the enzyme will be called a dehydrogenase.
     e. ***Tip***: MOST (but not all) dehydrogenases use NAD^+/NADH or FAD/$FADH_2$, regardless of the direction of the actual reaction (as many oxidation/reduction reactions are REVERSIBLE)

  2. For ***SYNTHETIC*** pathways, redox enzymes are named by:
     a. the **oxidized** molecule
     b. followed by <u>reductase</u>.
     c. ***Tip:*** MOST (but not all) reductases use $NADP^+$/NADPH, regardless of the direction of the actual reaction.

3. <u>Other exceptions</u>: The electron transport chain complexes have several names, some which also use the name <u>reductase</u>.

E. Other rules for naming enzymes
1. <u>Phosphatases</u> (classified—hydrolase)—hydrolyze off phosphate groups.

2. <u>Phosphorylases</u>—put phosphate groups on (classified—transferase).

3. <u>Mutases</u>—are isomerases that catalyze the **intra**molecular rearrangement of functional groups (i.e. in glycolysis, <u>phosphoglycerate</u> <u>mutase</u> moves a phosphate group from carbon 3 to carbon 2 of the molecule)

4. <u>Kinases</u> (classified--transferase)—transfers phosphate groups to/from ATP. Kinases are always named for the **molecule** that would be **accepting the phosphate group** from ATP. In other words, as if ATP is always the DONOR of the phosphate group.

   (1) Thus, if ATP is actually donating a phosphate group in a reaction (i.e. one of the substrates of the reaction)
       (i) Name the **SUBSTRATE** (the acceptor of the phosphate group)
       (ii) Followed by **kinase**
   (2) If ATP is a product of a reaction
       (i) Name the **PRODUCT** (the one that would be accepting the phosphate group from ATP if the reaction ran in the reverse direction)
       (ii) Followed by **kinase**
   (3) <u>For example</u>: in glycolysis there are 4 kinases:
       (i) In the first half of glycolysis (where ATP is used), the first two kinases are named for the **substrates** of the reactions: <u>hexo</u>kinase and <u>phosphofructo</u>kinase
       (ii) In the second half of glycolysis (where ATP is produced), the kinases are named for the **products** of the reactions: <u>phosphoglycerate</u> kinase and <u>pyruvate</u> kinase.

5. <u>Aminotransferase</u> (formerly called transaminase) [classified—transferase] transfers amino groups.
   (1) New nomenclature names the aminotransferase after the <u>donor</u> amino acid
   (2) Old nomenclature names the product amino acid first, then the product α-keto acid, followed by transaminase
   (3) Examples:
       (i) Rxn: alanine + α-ketoglutarate ↔ pyruvate + glutamate
            alanine aminotransferase (ALT)—new nomenclature
            glutamate/pyruvate transaminase (GPT)—old nomenclature
       (ii) (ii) Rxn: aspartate + α-ketoglutarate ↔ oxaloacetate + glutamate
            aspartate aminotransferase (AST)—new nomenclature

glutamate/oxaloacetate transaminase (GOT)—old nomenclature

(4) Clinical relevance: test for serum levels of these transaminases
  (i) liver damage → elevated levels of ALT and AST (example: old nomenclature may see as SGOT for "serum" GOT)

6. Hydrolase enzymes:
  (1) Name reactant
  (2) Plus attach **-ase** ending (ex. sucr<u>ase</u>--hydrolyzes sucrose)
  <u>Note</u>: Digestive enzymes are <u>hydrolases</u>

F. <u>NOTE</u>: There are often exceptions to these rules, but it is easier to note the exceptions when they occur, if one knows the general rules for naming enzymes.

Problem Set: Basic Principles of Oxidation States

IMPORTANT: Please do these problems and exercises by using your notes from this "oxidation states" chapter, which will provide more insight and comprehension than simply looking at the answers.

Figure 1.15: Exercise #1

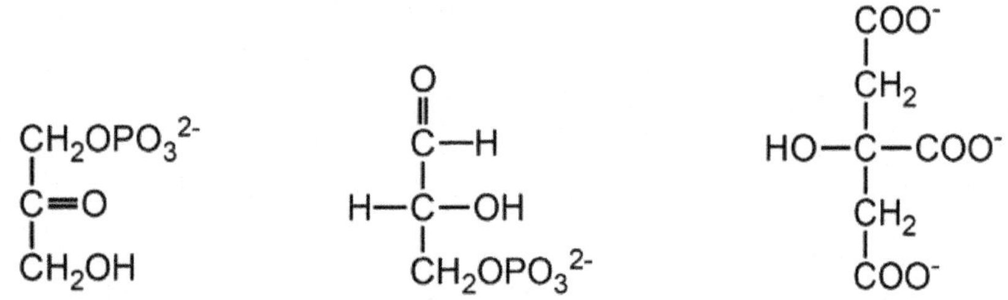

$CH_2OPO_3{}^{2-}$
|
$C=O$
|
CH_2OH

molecule 1

O
||
$C-H$
|
$H-C-OH$
|
$CH_2OPO_3{}^{2-}$

molecule 2

COO^-
|
CH_2
|
$HO-C-COO^-$
|
CH_2
|
COO^-

molecule 3

1. Which of the three molecules In **Figure 1.15** have functional groups that CANNOT be further oxidized? (Note, they all contain multiple functional groups, but which functional groups cannot be further oxidized)
   A. Molecule 1
   B. Molecule 2
   C. Molecule 3
   D. Molecules 1 and 3
   E. Molecules 1, 2, and 3

Figure 1.16: Exercise #2 and #3

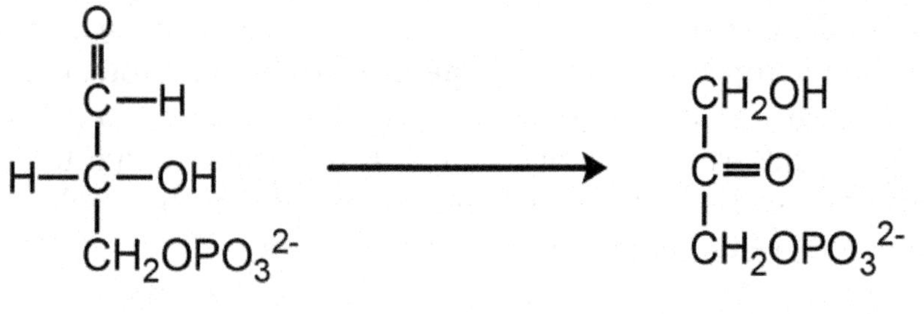

O
||
$C-H$
|
$H-C-OH$
|
$CH_2OPO_3{}^{2-}$

1

$\longrightarrow$

CH_2OH
|
$C=O$
|
$CH_2OPO_3{}^{2-}$

2

2. In the reaction drawn in **Figure 1.16**, what has happened to molecule 1 to convert it to molecule 2?
   A. Phosphorylation
   B. Dehydration
   C. Isomerization
   D. Oxidation
   E. Reduction

3. For the reaction drawn in **Figure 1.16**, what type of enzyme would carry out this reaction?

    A. Epimerase
    B. Isomerase
    C. Dehydrogenase
    D. Kinase
    E. Hydrolase

Figure 1.17: Exercise #4.

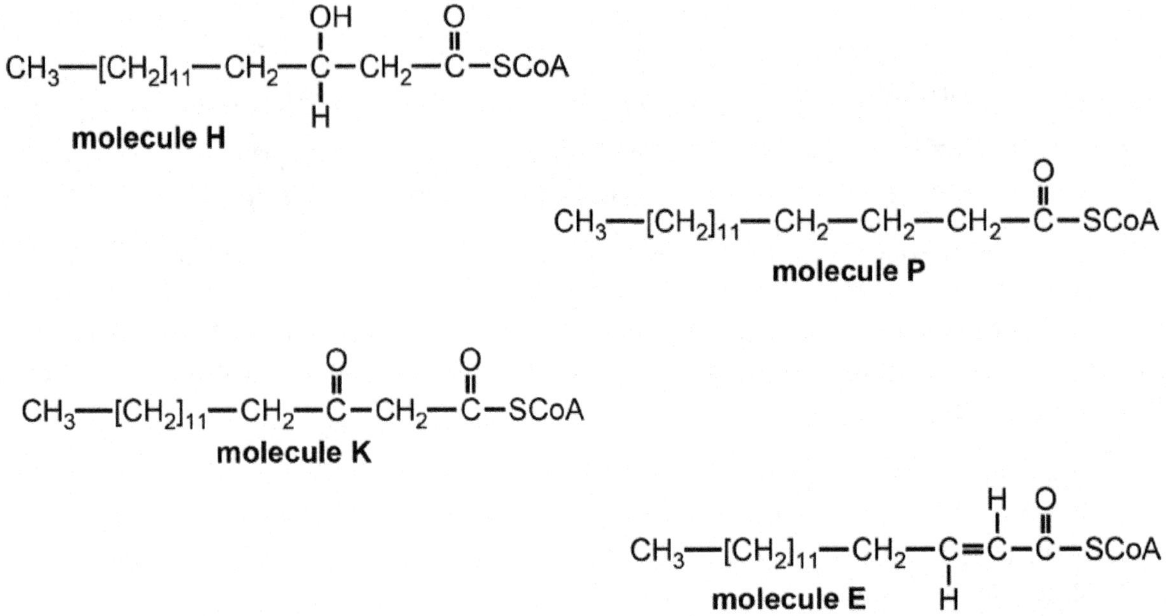

$$CH_3-[CH_2]_{11}-CH_2-\underset{\underset{H}{|}}{\overset{\overset{OH}{|}}{C}}-CH_2-\overset{\overset{O}{\|}}{C}-SCoA$$

molecule H

$$CH_3-[CH_2]_{11}-CH_2-CH_2-CH_2-\overset{\overset{O}{\|}}{C}-SCoA$$

molecule P

$$CH_3-[CH_2]_{11}-CH_2-\overset{\overset{O}{\|}}{C}-CH_2-\overset{\overset{O}{\|}}{C}-SCoA$$

molecule K

$$CH_3-[CH_2]_{11}-CH_2-\underset{\underset{H}{|}}{\overset{\overset{H}{|}}{C}}=C-\overset{\overset{O}{\|}}{C}-SCoA$$

molecule E

The four molecules have been "named" using random letters.

Exercise #4:

1. On a separate sheet of paper, re-draw the four molecules in **Figure 1.17** in the order in which a ***metabolic pathway*** would need to follow to go **from the most reduced molecule** (draw at the top of the page), **to the most oxidized molecule** (draw towards the bottom of the page). Leave space between the molecules to do the following steps. [HINT: Focus on the differences between the four molecules; and if the only difference between molecules is the number of hydrogens—then the molecule with <u>more hydrogens</u> is the <u>more reduced</u> molecule.]

2. Now draw reaction arrows between the molecules. (Since there are 4 molecules, you should draw three reaction arrows, indicating the three reactions that must take place to go from the most reduced molecule to the most oxidized molecule.) Now identify these three types of reactions (i.e. oxidation/reduction, etc.)

3. Now indicate the side reactants/products that are necessary for each of the three reactions.

4. Using the appropriate assigned molecule letter, name the enzyme that would carry out each of the three reactions. You need to know whether you are naming the enzyme for the reactant or product of the given reaction. Review the "Naming of Enzymes" section of the chapter—which provides some rules for how to name the enzymes. [For example: "molecule z dehydrogenase," as an enzyme that carries out an oxidation-reduction reaction. In this case, "molecule z" must be the <u>reduced</u> molecule in the reaction because that is how dehydrogenases are named.]

Figure 1.18: Exercise #5.

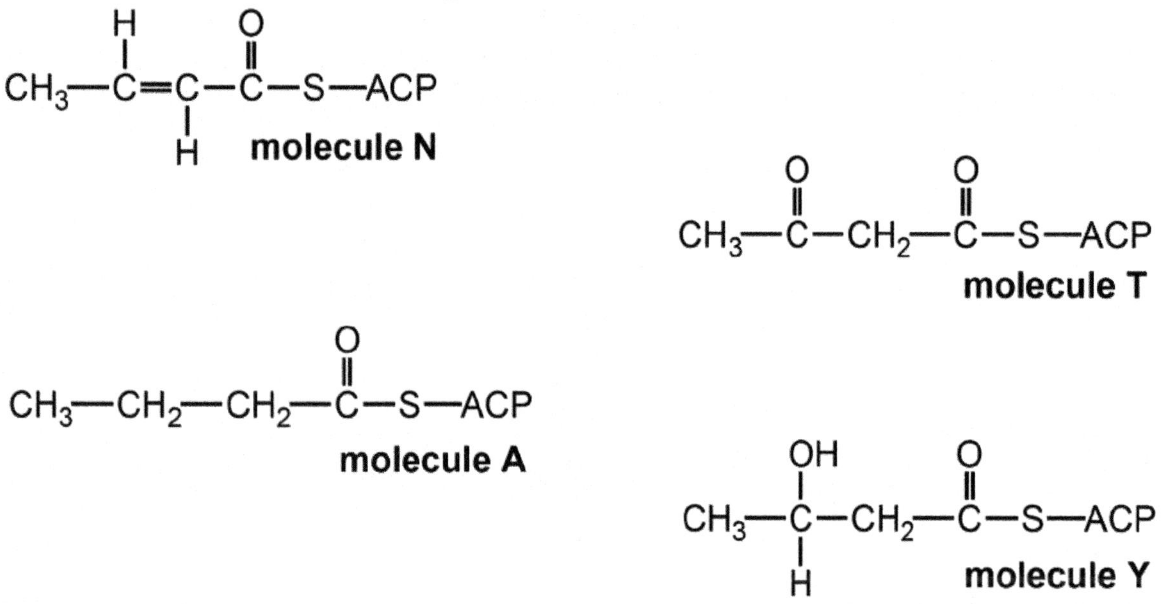

CH_3—C=C—C—S—ACP **molecule N**

CH_3—C—CH_2—C—S—ACP **molecule T**

CH_3—CH_2—CH_2—C—S—ACP **molecule A**

CH_3—C—CH_2—C—S—ACP **molecule Y**

The four molecules have been "named" using random letters.

Exercise #5:

1. On a separate sheet of paper, re-draw the four molecules in **Figure 1.18** in the order in which a ***metabolic pathway*** would need to follow to go **<u>from</u> the most oxidized molecule** (draw at the top of the page), **<u>to</u> the most reduced molecule** (draw towards the bottom of the page). Leave space between the molecules to do the following steps. [<u>HINT</u>: Focus on the differences between the four molecules; and if the only difference between molecules is the number of hydrogens—then the molecule with <u>more hydrogens</u> is the <u>more reduced</u> molecule.]

2. Now draw reaction arrows between the molecules. (Since there are 4 molecules, you should draw three reaction arrows, indicating the three reactions that must take place to go from the most oxidized molecule to the most reduced molecule.) Now identify these three types of reactions (i.e. oxidation/reduction, etc.)

3. Now indicate the side reactants/products that are necessary for each of the three reactions.

4. Using the appropriate assigned molecule letter, name the enzyme that would carry out each of the three reactions. You need to know whether you are naming the enzyme for the reactant or product of the given reaction. Review the "Naming of Enzymes" section—which provides some rules for how to name the enzymes. [For example: "molecule z reductase," as an enzyme that carries out an oxidation-reduction reaction. In this case, "molecule z" must be the <u>oxidized</u> molecule in the reaction because that is how reductases are named.]

Exercise #6:
Draw in the functional groups on the top carbons of molecules B, C, and D in **Figure 1.19** that would be required to convert molecule A to molecule E. [HINT: Again, focus on the differences between molecule A and molecule E.]

Figure 1.19: Exercise #6

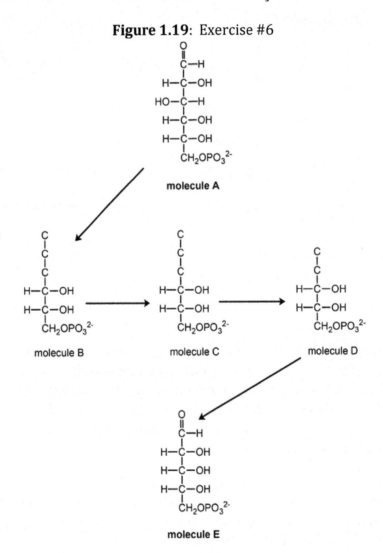

The four molecules have been "named" using random letters

Problem Set: Solutions

1. (D) Molecule 1 has a ketone functionality and Molecule 3 has a 3° alcohol functionality, neither of which can be further oxidized.

2. (C) Isomerization of an aldehyde to a ketone.

3. (B) Isomerase

Exercise #4: (see **Figure 1.20**)
For reactions 1 and 3: Oxidation and reduction reactions are ALWAYS coupled. However, by labeling reactions 1 and 3 as oxidation reactions, the reactions are referring to what is happening in going from molecule P to molecule E (reaction 1) and molecule H to molecule K (reaction 3). Again, focus on what is DIFFERENT about each of these molecules. Many molecules have more than one functional group—one needs to recognize what is changing about the molecules in the reactions to figure out what type of reaction is happening, and the type of enzyme that will carry out the reaction.

In reaction 1, carbons 2 and 3 of molecule P are at the level of an alkane. In molecule E, there is a double bond between carbons 2 and 3. Therefore, the molecule has been oxidized to form molecule E. Thus, something must be reduced. FAD is typically used when oxidizing something from the level of an alkane to an alkene. So FAD is reduced to $FADH_2$. Enzymes that carry out oxidation-reduction reactions in generally "catabolic" pathways (i.e. going "down" the oxidation chart) are dehydrogenases—which are named for the more REDUCED molecule. Molecule P (alkane level) is the more reduced molecule of the two, so the enzyme name is "molecule P" dehydrogenase.

Reaction 2 is a hydration of the alkene of molecule E to form molecule H. This is not an oxidation reaction. It is simply a hydration, the addition of H_2O across the double bond—hence H_2O is a second reactant necessary for this reaction. This enzyme name would not be obvious because there are no "hard and fast" rules for naming enzymes that carry out hydration and dehydration reactions. However, these enzymes are typically named in some fashion after the molecule that is being hydrated (hydratase) or dehydrated (dehydratase)—though these are typically reversible reactions. In this case, the reaction is hydrating molecule E. So the enzyme is called "molecule E" hydratase.

In reaction 3, carbon 3 of molecule H has an alcohol group (-OH group) on it. Molecule K has a keto- group on carbon 3. Thus this reaction is also an oxidation reaction (a.k.a. dehydrogenation). NAD^+ is typically used for the oxidations of secondary alcohols to ketones (and for oxidations of primary alcohols to aldehydes, as well as aldehydes oxidized to carboxylic acids). Thus, NAD^+ is reduced to NADH + H^+. Again, the enzyme would be a dehydrogenase named for the more REDUCED molecule. The alcohol group of molecule H is more reduced than the keto-group on molecule K (again focus on the differences between molecules). Thus, the enzyme would be "molecule H" dehydrogenase.

Figure 1.20: Exercise #4 solution

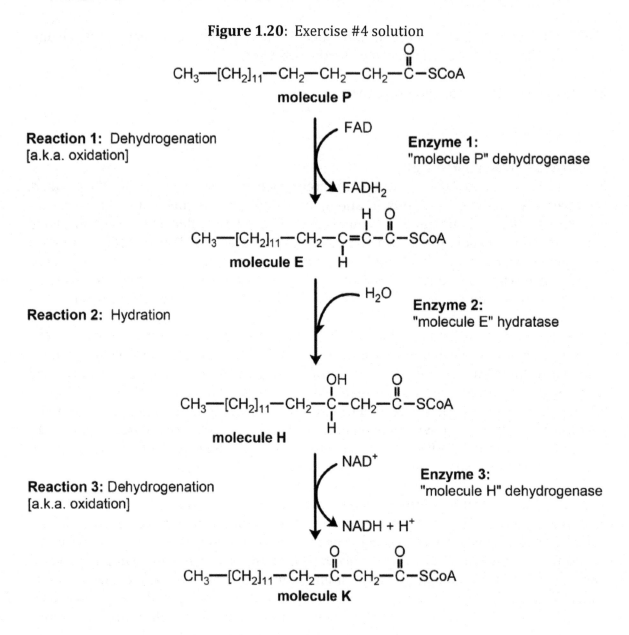

Exercise #5: (see **Figure 1.21**)

For reactions 1 and 3: Oxidation and reduction reactions are ALWAYS coupled. However, by labeling reactions 1 and 3 as reduction reactions, the reactions are referring to what is happening in going from molecule T to molecule Y (reaction 1) and molecule N to molecule A (reaction 3). Again, focus on what is DIFFERENT about each of these molecules. Many molecules have more than one functional group—one needs to recognize what is changing about the molecules in the reactions to figure out what type of reaction is happening, and the type of enzyme that will carry out the reaction.

In reaction 1, Molecule T has a ketone group on carbon 3, while carbon 3 of molecule Y has an alcohol group (-OH group or hydroxy group) on it. Thus this reaction is a reduction reaction, and something must also be oxidized. NADPH + H$^+$ is typically used for <u>all</u> reduction reactions in synthetic pathways. Thus, NADPH + H$^+$ is oxidized to NADP$^+$. The enzyme would be a reductase named for the more OXIDIZED molecule. The ketone group of molecule T is more oxidized than the hydroxy group on molecule Y (again focus on the differences between molecules). Thus, the enzyme would be "molecule T" reductase.

Reaction 2 is a dehydration removing the hydroxy group of molecule Y to form the alkene of molecule N. This is not an oxidation-reduction reaction. It is simply a dehydration reaction, the removal of H$_2$O to form the double bond (recall alcohols and alkenes are at the same oxidation level). This enzyme name would not be obvious because there are no "hard and fast" rules for naming enzymes that carry out hydration and dehydration reactions. However, these enzymes are typically named in some fashion after the molecule that is being hydrated (hydratase) or dehydrated (dehydratase)—though these are typically reversible reactions. In this case, the reaction is dehydrating molecule Y. So the enzyme is called "molecule Y" dehydratase.

In reaction 3, molecule N has a double bond between carbons 2 and 3, while both carbons 2 and 3 of molecule A are at the level of an alkane. Therefore, molecule N has been reduced to form molecule A. Thus, something must also be oxidized. NADPH + H$^+$ is typically used for <u>all</u> reduction reactions in synthetic pathways. Thus, NADPH + H$^+$ is oxidized to NADP$^+$. The enzyme would be a reductase named for the more OXIDIZED molecule. The alkene group of molecule N is more oxidized than the alkane carbons on molecule A (again focus on the differences between molecules). Thus, the enzyme would be "molecule N" reductase.

Figure 1.21: Exercise #5 solution

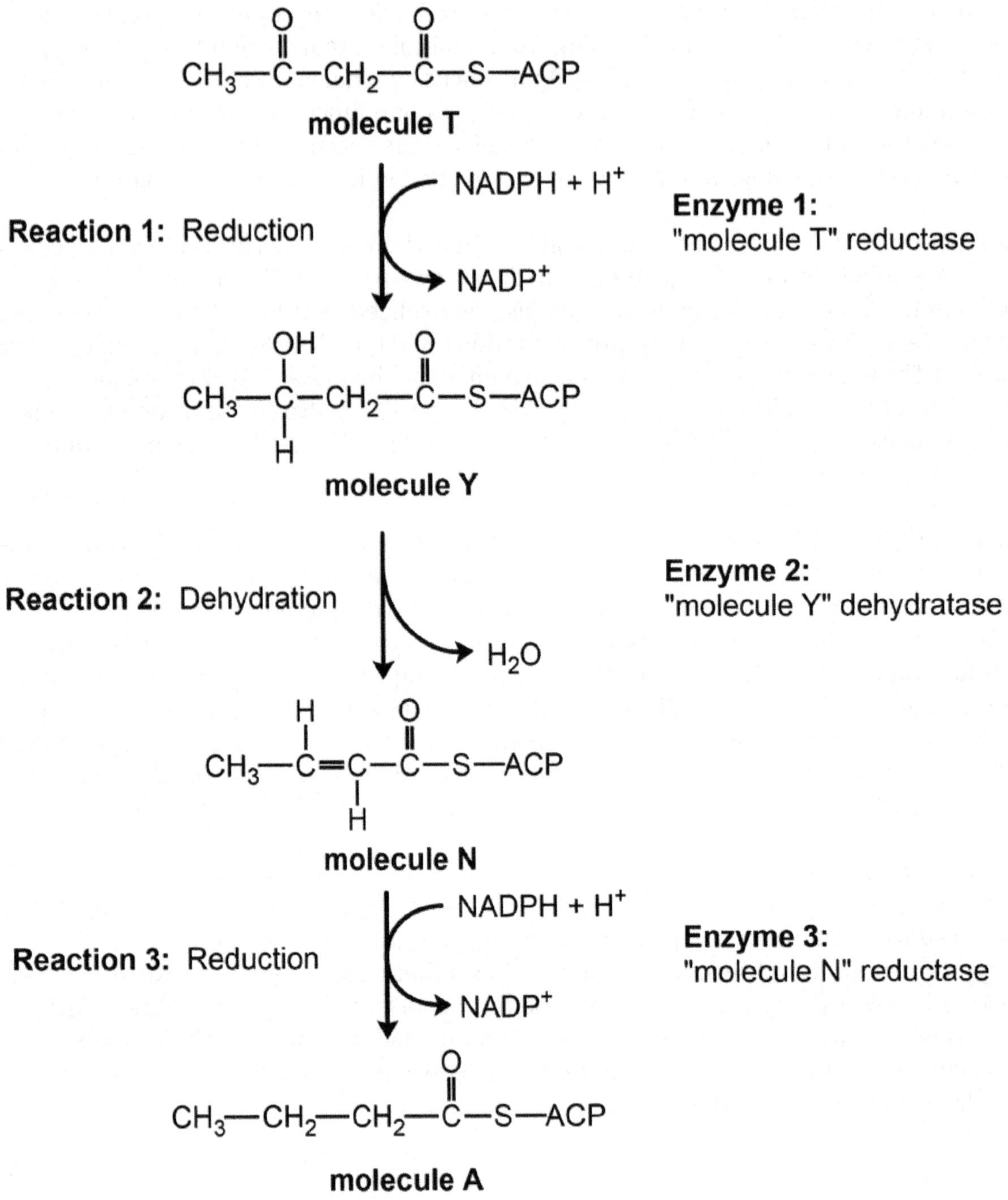

Exercise #6 solution: (see **Figure 1.22**)

There are several possibilities for the solution to this problem (one possibility is illustrated in **Figure 1.22**). The primary differences one needs to notice between molecules A and E is that carbon #1 of molecule A is removed and that carbon #2 of molecule E, which was carbon #3 of molecule A, has the –OH group pointing in the opposite direction. (Yes, the orientation of functional groups around chiral carbons is significant.)

The two main reactions one needs to include are the oxidation of the aldehyde carbon #1 of molecule A to a carboxylic acid group, and the oxidation of an –OH group on either carbon #2 or carbon #3 of molecule A to a keto group (creating either an α-keto acid or a β-keto acid).

While generally in metabolism the oxidation to the acid would occur first, for this exercise it does not matter which oxidation one put first—just as long as both oxidations were included.

If one chose to make an α-keto acid, molecule D would have been an aldose after the decarboxylation. However, carbon #2 would have the –OH in the wrong configuration—thus an epimerase would be needed to convert molecule D to molecule E.

If one chose to make a β-keto acid as shown in **Figure 1.22** (preferred metabolically because β-keto acids are easier to decarboxylate,), molecule D would be a ketose after the decarboxylation and an isomerase would be needed to convert molecule D to molecule E.

Figure 1.22: Exercise #6 solution

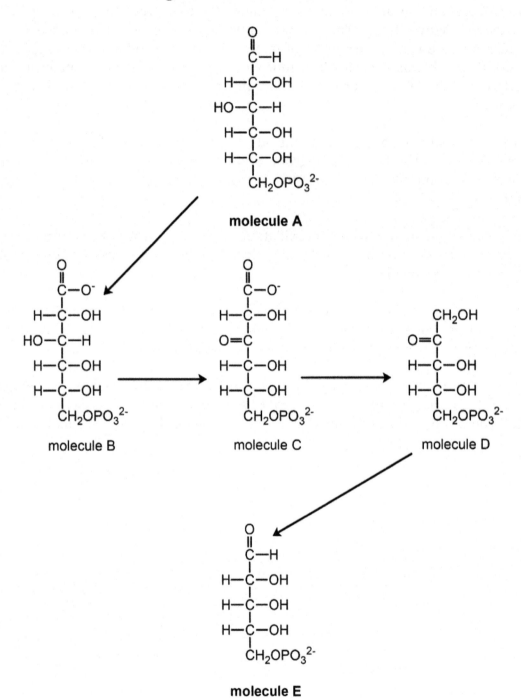

CHAPTER 2: METABOLISM OVERVIEW AND GLYCOLYSIS

Objectives:

1. Define the process of glycolysis.
2. Explain the purpose of the pathway of glycolysis.
   a. Account for the net yield of ATP in the catabolism of glucose to pyruvate; which reactions use and which reactions produce ATP.
3. Identify where glycolysis takes place in the cell.
4. Explain how glycolysis is carried out in the cell.
   a. Name and recognize the structures of the starting materials, key intermediates, end products.
   b. Name the enzymes involved in the aerobic and anaerobic catabolism of glucose and identify the reactions they catalyze.
   c. Identify the types of glycolytic reactions that are carried out by kinases and dehydrogenases (and how they are named), isomerases, mutases, aldolase and enolase.
   d. Describe the purpose of the glucose to glucose 6-P reaction, and identify the two isozymes that carry out this reaction.
   e. Describe the purpose of the last three steps (steps 8, 9, and 10) of glycolysis in   regards to producing the end products ATP and pyruvate.
   f. Define the term "substrate level phosphorylation", and identify the intermediates and reactions of glycolysis that fit this definition.
5. Explain when glycolysis takes place.
   a. Identify the major regulatory steps in glycolysis, the enzymes that catalyze these steps, and the molecules that regulate them.
   b. Identify the key reaction that differentiates aerobic from anaerobic glycolysis, and why oxygen availability controls whether or not this additional reaction is carried out.
6. Identify the fates of each of the products of glycolysis, under both aerobic and anaerobic conditions.
   a. Describe the difference in how cytosolic NAD^+ is regenerated for glyceraldehyde 3-P dehydrogenase during aerobic versus anaerobic glycolysis.

    b. Identify the link between glyceraldehyde 3-P dehydrogenase and lactate dehydrogenase during anaerobic glycolysis.

    c. Describe why shuttles are necessary to carry the electrons via hydrogens (reducing equivalents) between the cytoplasm and the mitochondria under aerobic conditions, and list the two different types of shuttles.

7. Describe the physiological role for the different affinities for glucose (K_m values), rates (V_{max} values), and regulation for glucokinase versus hexokinase.

OVERVIEW OF METABOLISM

There are four major classes of biological molecules (see **Table 2.1**): carbohydrates (or sugars), lipids, proteins, and nucleic acids (DNA and RNA). These large "functioning biomolecules" are polymers or are "polymer-like" and are made from monomers termed "basic building blocks." Glycogen is a polymer of glucose monomers. Proteins are polymers made up of amino acid monomers. DNA and RNA are polymers made up of nucleotide monomers. Triacylglycerols (a.k.a. triacylglycerides or triglycerides) are "polymer-like." A triacylglycerol has three fatty acid "monomers" attached to a glycerol backbone.

The ability to attach the basic building blocks together to make these larger functioning biomolecules requires energy, and usually reducing power in the form of NADPH. Thus, the synthesis of these functioning biomolecules generally goes through an "activated precursor" stage, which harnesses the energy needed to create bonds between the basic building blocks. For instance, monosaccharides are typically attached to UTP to form a UDP-sugar (i.e. UDP-glucose). The removal of the UDP unit provides the energy for the attachment of the sugar to the larger molecule (as in the synthesis of glycogen or a glycolipid).

Table 2.1: Four classes of biomolecules

FUNCTIONING BIOMOLECULE	ACTIVATED PRECURSOR	BASIC BUILDING BLOCK
1. Carbohydrate [i.e. glycogen]	UDP-glucose	Monosaccharide
2. Lipids (Fat) [i.e. TAGs and cholesterol]	Fatty acyl-CoA	Fatty acids
3. Proteins	tRNA-amino acid	amino acids
4. Nucleic acids [i.e. DNA and RNA]	dNTPs and NTPs	ribo- (and deoxyribo-) nucleic acids

The metabolic pathways described in this text will focus on catabolism (breakdown) and anabolism (synthesis) of the "monomers" or "basic building blocks" themselves. In particular, the focus will be on the pathways associated with the catabolism and synthesis of glucose and fatty acids. The nutrients one obtains in the diet are broken down to these basic building blocks and ultimately absorbed by various tissues. These basic building blocks can be catabolized further by cells or used for other synthetic processes. The body also has the ability to make some of these basic building blocks *de novo* (i.e. "from scratch" in the cells).

HOW TO STUDY METABOLIC PATHWAYS

When one is describing an event to someone else, there are generally six key questions one should answer to relay the complete story of the event: Who? What? Why? Where? When? How? Answering these six questions is also essential in developing an understanding of metabolic pathways.

The question "who?" is referring to what organism is being studied. For this text, the answer to "who?" is humans, but many of the pathways covered are found in other animals, plants and microorganisms. Bacteria inhabit nearly every environmental niche on earth. As these bacteria are exposed to temperatures, pH, and nutrients unique to their environments, bacteria can catalyze many different types of reaction that humans cannot do within their normal temperature and pH ranges. However, bacteria still have to carry out many of the basic types of reaction sequences needed for the catabolism and anabolism of their functioning biomolecules.

All pathways in this text will provide an answer to four of the basic questions: what, why, where, and how. The question "what" refers to the definition of the pathway. The question "why" is the purpose or function of the pathway. "Where" describes where the pathway takes place in a cell and/or which tissue(s). Some pathways only take place, for instance, in the liver. Ketone body synthesis is an example of a pathway that only takes place in the liver. "How" is a question that seems to encompass everything else regarding the reactions, mechanisms, etc. of a pathway. There are key points, though, that one should know about how a pathway occurs that will help keep a "big picture" perspective on what the pathway needs to accomplish. Learning key structures of pathways will help one form a "picture" in one's mind of the overall sequence of the pathway. By learning how pathways follow the basic recipe of metabolism, then one can simply learn the "list" of the reaction sequences. If one truly understands how to apply these general patterns and rules, one can draw out or recognize any step based on their knowledge of key structures, oxidation state sequences, and enzyme naming rules.

In beginning to understand "how" the pathway occurs, start with knowing the starting and ending products of the pathway, including their structures. This is the "picture" of what the pathway is starting with and trying to get to. Know any steps that make or require ATP, as these are often important steps of a pathway. Know the vitamins and coenzymes necessary for particular enzymes. Coenzymes are typically derived from vitamins. Patients suffering from particular vitamin deficiencies display clinical signs and symptoms based on the enzymes affected.

The question "when" will be answered as one begins to understand how various metabolic pathways fit together. The answer to the question "when" demonstrates one's understanding of the integration of metabolic pathways. Answering the question "when" for a particular pathway includes indicating: under what conditions should the pathway be on (active) or off (inhibited); the enzymes that are regulated for the pathway and what regulates them—their activators and/or inhibitors; what other pathways need to run simultaneously or in sequence; and what pathways will never be "on" in the *same cell* at the same time. Answers to the question "when" will be provided in the context of the pathways covered. However, answering the question "when" is a continual process. As one learns more pathways and the complexities involved in regulation of them all, the understanding of "when" (i.e. the integration of metabolism) is more challenging.

KEY STRUCTURES TO BE ABLE TO DRAW AND RECOGNIZE

To learn structures of metabolic pathways, there are key structures one should know—both to be able to draw them and to recognize them. **Figure 2.1** indicates _some_ of these key structures that will aide in identifying other structures of carbohydrate metabolism. These structures include glycerol, acetone, pyruvate, and the linear and cyclical forms of glucose and fructose. *Note* that the proper three letter abbreviation for glucose is "**glc**," not glu (as many texts use). The three letter abbreviation for the amino acid glutamate is "glu." It is confusing to use the same three letter abbreviation for both molecules. This text will use the abbreviation "glc" for glucose.

For example, if one knows the structure of glucose and fructose, one does not need to memorize the structures for the first three steps of glycolysis. The names of the molecules for these first three steps are glucose, glucose 6-phosphate, fructose 6-phosphate, and fructose 1,6-bisphosphate. If one knows the structures of glucose and fructose and how the carbons are numbered, one knows where to put phosphate groups based on the names of the structures. Now it is okay to simply learn the order of the reactions, especially when one understands how the enzymes that carry out the reactions are named.

Figure 2.1: Key structures to know.

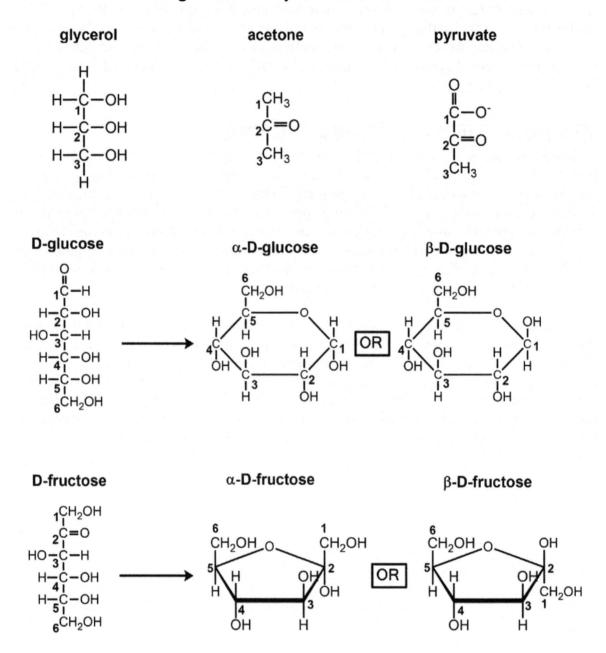

Be able to draw and recognize them.

GLYCOLYSIS

As mentioned previously, every metabolic pathway covered in this text will answer four key questions that one should understand for a given pathway: What? Why? Where? How? Glycolysis, as the first pathway covered, will begin to apply the principles that were introduced in the oxidation states chapter. Particular aspects of the regulation of glycolysis will be covered to establish certain overarching concepts of metabolic regulation, and to indicate some of the complexity involved in regulation of even a single pathway.

The overall reaction of aerobic glycolysis, shown in **Figure 2.2**, catabolizes a molecule of glucose to yield 2 pyruvate, 2 ATP, 2 NADH, 2 protons and 2 water molecules. For anaerobic glycolysis, the same net yield of ATP is produced, but there is no net NADH formed. NADH is still formed at the same step, but it is utilized differently because the electrons from it cannot go to the mitochondria.

Figure 2.2: Net reaction of glycolysis under aerobic and anaerobic conditions

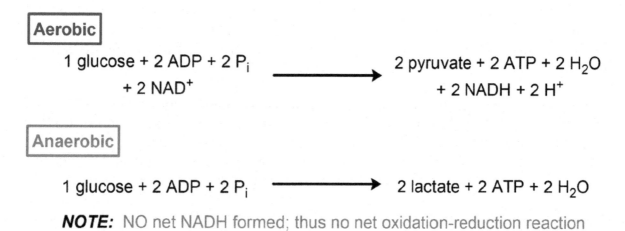

To define the pathway of glycolysis (i.e. What?): glycolysis is the catabolism of glucose, (a six carbon molecule) to two pyruvates (three carbon molecules) under aerobic conditions; or to two lactates (three carbon molecules) under anaerobic conditions.

The purpose of glycolysis (i.e. Why?) is to produce ATP directly, reducing power in the form of NADH, and molecules of carbon dioxide (CO_2) for the excretion of carbons. Note that the structure of glucose has no phosphates on it and pyruvate has no phosphates on it. However, this pathway will generate ATP, which is requires phosphorylation reactions. This pathway will put phosphates on intermediates and then use them to phosphorylate ADP to make ATP. By the end of the glycolytic pathway, no carbons will be lost, but two out of the six carbons will be ready to be removed. Recall the goal is to get to carbons oxidized to carboxylic acids, but carboxylic acid groups are stable. To get a carboxylic acid group to leave, a keto group needs to be placed nearby in either the alpha or beta position. For a three carbon molecule the keto group must be at the alpha position. Creating a beta keto acid is not possible, because the beta carbon is an end carbon on pyruvate, which would be an aldehyde group. What happens to the reducing power, NADH, formed will differentiate aerobic versus anaerobic glycolysis.

Glycolysis occurs in the cytosol of the cell (Where?). Most catabolic processes occur in the mitochondria, as a purpose of catabolism is to generate ATP from the breakdown of nutrients. The reducing power generated goes to the electron transport chain (ETC) for ATP production from oxidative phosphorylation. However, glycolysis is the only *catabolic* pathway that generates ATP from ADP from nutrient breakdown that does not depend on the mitochondria. [Note: ATP can certainly be made from *de novo* synthesis of nucleotides, but catabolic pathways produce chemical energy by phosphorylating a ribonucleoside diphosphate (i.e. ADP) to a ribonucleoside triphosphate (i.e. ATP).] This is why it is so important that the glycolytic pathway is not located in the mitochondria. If the electron transport chain is not working, due to lack of oxygen, glycolysis becomes the only catabolic ATP producing pathway via anaerobic glycolysis. As an example, mature red blood cells have no mitochondria. Mature red blood cells can only produce ATP by anaerobic glycolysis. The purpose of a red blood cell is to deliver oxygen to the tissues. Mitochondria are the organelles that use the most oxygen, as oxygen is the final electron acceptor of the electron transport chain. It makes sense that a mature red blood cell does not have mitochondria, so it does not use what it is trying to deliver. Otherwise a red blood cell would use the oxygen itself.

The details of the individual reactions of glycolysis (How?) will be covered in this chapter. Important key concepts to know include the starting and ending product structures, structures of key intermediates, the committed step reaction, and the enzymes and reactions the produce the end products. One should also know the regulated enzymes and what regulates them for the reactions that they carry out.

Figure 2.3 shows the entire glycolytic pathway with the names of the intermediates and enzymes, though the molecular structures are not shown. The 10 reactions of glycolysis are numbered. The key to point out in this overview figure, which will be reiterated, is what happens to the molecules of NADH formed in the glyceraldehyde 3-phosphate dehydrogenase step. Under conditions where the mitochondria are functional (aerobic conditions), the cell wants to shuttle the electrons, carried by the hydride ion, in the mitochondria to be used to make ATP by the electron transport chain. Shuttles move the electrons carried by the hydride into the mitochondria and, in the process, regenerate cytosolic NAD+ for the glyceraldehyde 3-phosphate dehydrogenase reaction.

Under anaerobic conditions the electron transport chain is not working. Under these conditions the electrons from this NADH cannot be shuttled into the mitochondria. However, glycolysis will stop, as well, if cells do not have a means of regenerating cytosolic NAD+ for the glyceraldehyde 3-phosphate dehydrogenase step. Therefore, the purpose of the pyruvate to lactate conversion (see **Figure 2.3**) by lactate dehydrogenase is the regeneration cytosolic NAD^+ under anaerobic conditions. The cell can continue to do glycolysis and to produce ATP. Thus, the key difference between aerobic and anaerobic glycolysis is what happens to the NADH generated by the glyceraldehyde 3-phosphate dehydrogenase step.

Figure 2.3: The glycolytic pathway

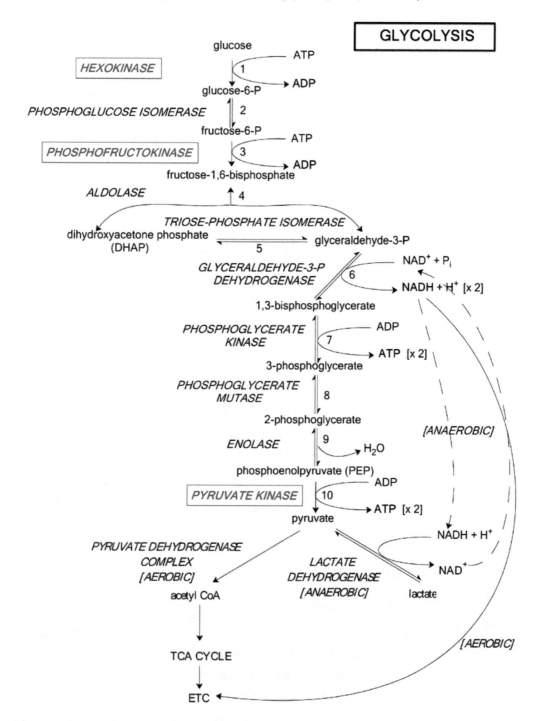

Figure 2.4: The first five steps of glycolysis

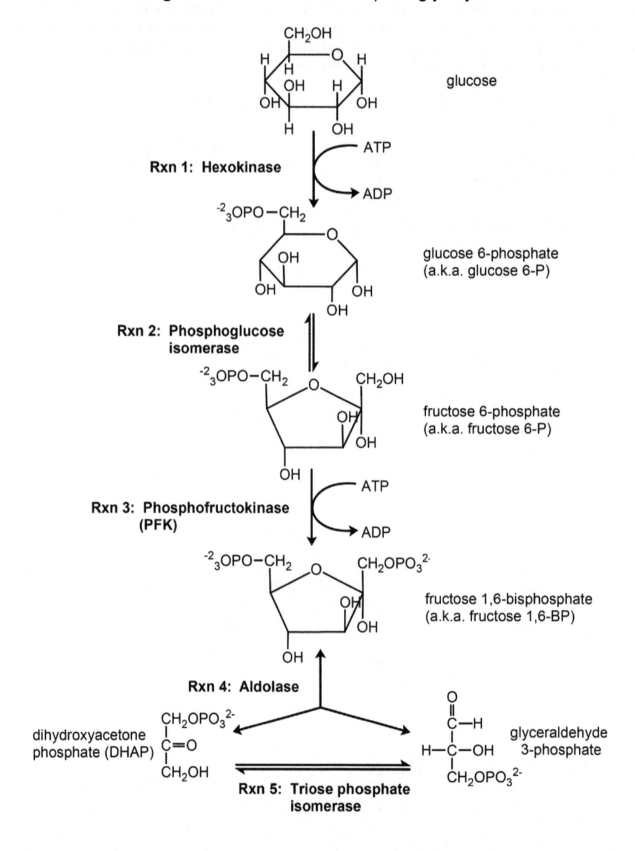

Figure 2.4 shows the first five steps of glycolysis with the structures. Each of the reactions of glycolysis will be covered step-by-step, but this figure shows the first half of glycolysis drawn in sequence. In covering the details of the reactions, "reasons" will be presented to help one think about "why" the reactions must be carried out in a particular order. The reactions shown in the oxidation states flow chart (**Figure 1.7**) present the pattern of the oxidation of carbon atoms, but there are other reaction types that need to occur in a cell. The objective in presenting these "reasons" is to help one remember the order that reactions need to occur, especially when the pathways include reactions not included in the oxidation states flow chart. The method for how the enzymes are named will also be covered.

The first reaction of glycolysis is shown in **Figure 2.5**, which phosphorylates glucose to form glucose 6-phosphate. Glucose is shown with its six carbons numbered appropriately. If you compare and contrast glucose to glucose 6-phosphate, the reaction put a phosphate group on glucose at carbon #6. The phosphate group comes from ATP. This is a catabolic pathway, but to get it started the cell will need to use a little bit ATP. The investment of some energy to start the pathway ensures the cell needs to do the pathway. Most catabolic pathways do require an input of energy in the beginning.

Figure 2.5: REACTION 1–Phosphorylation of glucose (glc) at carbon #6 using ATP

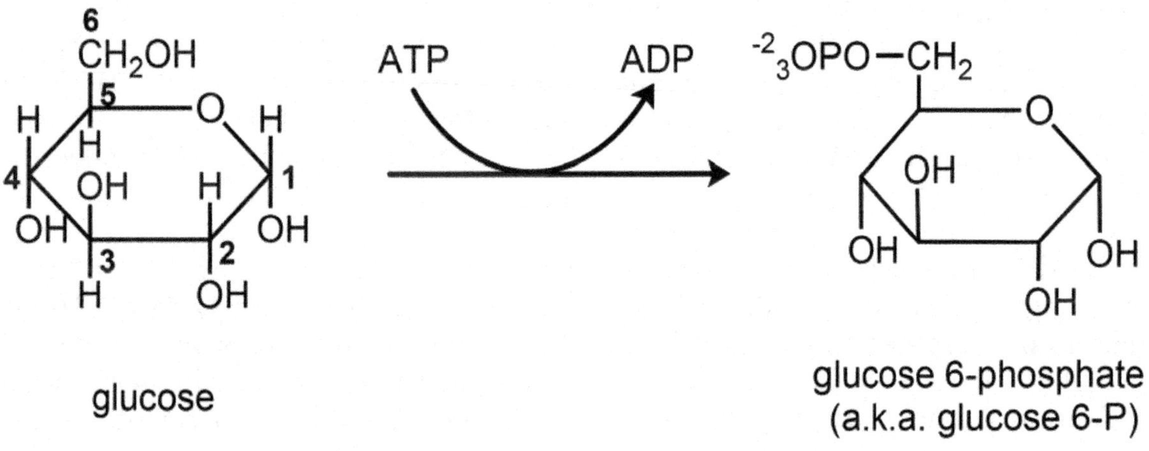

glucose

glucose 6-phosphate
(a.k.a. glucose 6-P)

Enzyme: hexokinase (or glucokinase, an isozyme)

Kinases are enzymes that transfer a phosphate group to a molecule, usually from ATP. Kinases are named for the molecule that accepts the phosphate from ATP. Therefore one would expect this enzyme to be called glucose kinase, or "in short"—***glucokinase***. Glucokinase is an isozyme form of the enzyme catalyzing this reaction in certain tissues. However, the enzyme that carries out this reaction in all cells is called ***hexokinase***. Hexoses are six-carbon sugars. The suffix "-ose" is used in molecular names to indicate a sugar (a.k.a. carbohydrate). Hexokinase is an enzyme that can phosphorylate other six-carbon sugars such as fructose and mannose, although it has a high affinity for glucose.

Isozymes are different forms of an enzyme, encoded by different genes, that have the same general architecture and catalytic mechanism, but they are regulated differently. Hexokinase and glucokinase are isozymes. They both catalyze glucose + ATP to glucose 6-phosphate + ADP. Hexokinase is in all tissues of the body, while glucokinase is in the liver and islet cells of the pancreas. The K_m for hexokinase is low (0.1 mM) compared to the K_m for glucokinase (10 mM), which means hexokinase has a higher affinity for glucose than glucokinase. The V_{max} for hexokinase is also low relative to the V_{max} for glucokinase. The purpose for these differences is that the liver allows the glucose coming from the diet via portal circulation from the small intestine to pass through to ensure the blood glucose is maintained at about 5 mM. Once the blood glucose begins to rise past 5 mM, the hepatocytes (i.e. liver cells) begin to take up the excess glucose and quickly phosphorylate it to glucose 6-phosphate. Thus the liver ensures that all other tissues have first access to glucose to use it and replenish their own glucose stores, if necessary.

Hexokinase is a regulated enzyme, and is inhibited by high cellular concentrations of glucose 6-phosphate. Glucokinase is also *not* inhibited by high cellular concentrations of glucose 6-phosphate. When cells have enough glucose, the glucose 6-phosphate concentration is high and inhibits hexokinase. Inhibition of hexokinase leads to inhibition of glucose uptake into the cell. Glucokinase cannot be inhibited by glucose 6-phosphate because the liver must take up all the excess glucose coming in via portal circulation to prevent blood glucose concentrations from becoming too high, leading to hyperglycemia. The liver cells can use the glucose to replenish their ATP levels, their glycogen stores, and if there is still excess glucose coming in—the liver cells convert it to fat (a.k.a. triacylglycerides).

This reaction is irreversible. An irreversible reaction is a reaction in which the Gibbs free energy of the reaction under cellular conditions (typically indicated as ΔG or $\Delta G'$) is equal to or more negative than -4 kcal/mol (-16.74 kJ/mol). In these cases, the cell generally cannot manipulate the concentration of products to reactants in the equation for ΔG to make the reaction go in the reverse direction. Under cellular conditions, the reaction catalyzed by hexokinase is even more favorable ($\Delta G \approx$ -8 kcal/mol) than under biochemical standard conditions ($\Delta G^{o'}$ = -4 kcal/mol). One can think of the irreversibility of the hexokinase reaction in another manner. The Gibbs free energy under biochemical standard conditions ($\Delta G^{o'}$) of the cleavage of a phosphoanhydride bond of ATP would yield approximately -7.3 kcal/mol. To reverse this reaction and phosphorylate ADP to make a phosphoanhydride bond of ATP, the cleavage of a phosphate group on carbon #6 would have yield more than -7.3 kcal/mol (as some energy is always lost as heat). The $\Delta G^{o'}$ of cleavage of an alcohol phosphate bond, such as this one, would only provide about -3 kcal/mol. Thus, an alcohol phosphate would not have enough energy in the bond to catalyze the reverse reaction, which would make a molecule of ATP.

The phosphorylation of glucose as glucose 6-phosphate traps the glucose inside the cell. When glucose enters the cell through specific glucose transport proteins, some of which are hormonally regulated, glucose immediately gets phosphorylated and cannot go back across the cellular membrane. Cells take up glucose molecules for "their own use." Only the liver and kidneys have the enzyme glucose 6-phosphatase that can clip off the phosphate group from glucose 6-phosphate to form glucose, which can be released back into the blood.

The reaction catalyzed by hexokinase is *not* the "committed step" of glycolysis. A "committed step" is the reaction of a pathway in which the product of that reaction is constrained to proceed through the remainder of the pathway. Glucose 6-phosphate, though, is an intermediate for other pathways. Glucose 6-phosphate is a key branch point between several pathways such as glycogen synthesis, glycogen breakdown, the pentose phosphate pathway, or the formation of glucose from gluconeogenesis in specific tissues (i.e. the liver and kidneys).

There is a particular rationale one can think of to understand the sequence of the first three steps of glycolysis. For these first steps of glycolysis, the goal is to phosphorylate the two end carbons of glucose (#1 and #6), but only if these carbons have a primary alcohol group. This first reaction does phosphorylate carbon #6, which has a primary alcohol. Carbon #1, the other end carbon of glucose, does not have a primary alcohol. This is more obvious when glucose is drawn in its straight chain form (see **Figure 2.6**), in which one can see that carbon #1 of glucose is an aldehyde. The cell wants to phosphorylate it, though, as a primary alcohol. Recall from the oxidation states flow chart (**Figure 1.7**) that an aldehyde can be isomerized to a ketone, and both are at the same oxidation state. If one knows the structure of glucose (an aldose or aldehyde sugar) and fructose (a ketose or keto sugar), one can draw this reaction, which is shown in **Figure 2.6**. Notice that in the molecule of fructose 6-phosphate, carbon #1 now has a primary alcohol. This is the purpose of reaction 2 of glycolysis: the isomerization of glucose 6-phosphate to fructose 6-phosphate to produce carbon #1 with a primary alcohol functionality. This primary alcohol will then be phosphorylated in the reaction #3 of glycolysis.

Reaction 2 isomerizes glucose 6-phosphate to fructose 6-phosphate, and both the cyclical and the linear structures are shown in **Figure 2.6**. Both molecules still have a phosphate group on carbon #6. In the cyclical structures, glucose 6-phosphate has a pyranose ring (a 6-membered ring). Fructose 6-phosphate has a furanose ring (a 5-membered ring). The isomerization of these two molecules is readily reversible. This is an isomerization reaction and, therefore, the enzyme that catalyzes it is an isomerase. There are no definitive rules for naming isomerases. In this case, the enzyme is named after the substrate. One could call the enzyme glucose 6-phosphate isomerase, but the enzyme name drops the six and puts the "phospho" in front to call it ***phosphoglucose isomerase***, or more often simply known as ***phosphoglucoisomerase***.

Figure 2.6: REACTION 2–Isomerization of Glc-6-P to Fructose 6-P.

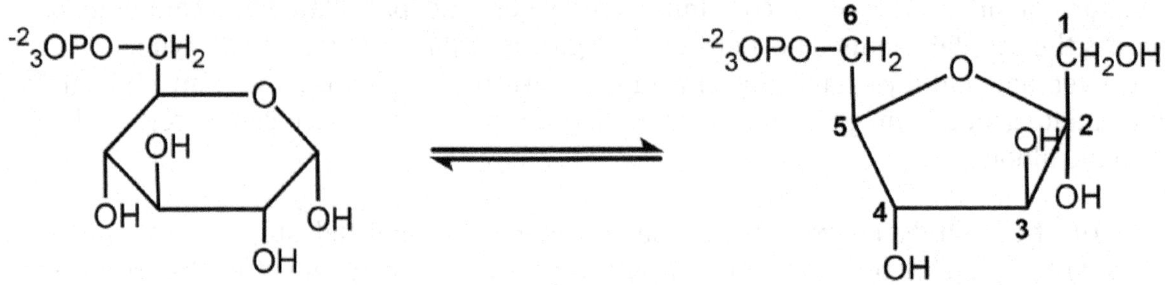

glucose 6-P

6-membered pyranose ring

fructose 6-phosphate
(a.k.a. fructose 6-P)

5-membered furanose ring

**Enzyme: phosphoglucoisomerase
(a.k.a. phosphoglucose isomerase)**

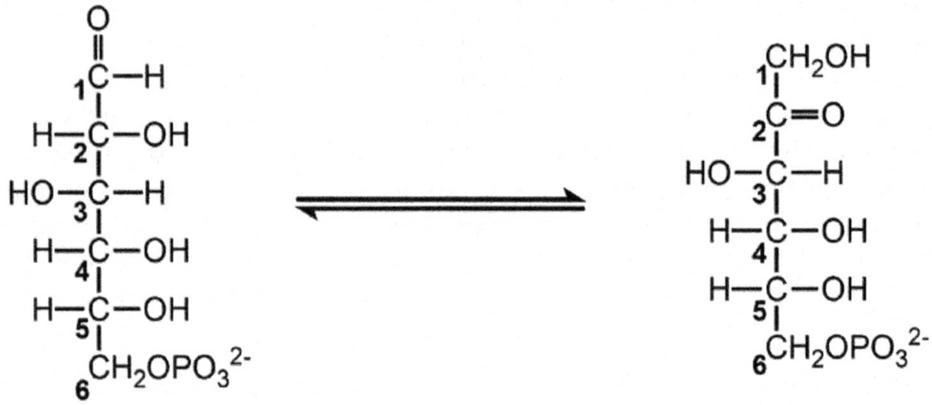

glucose 6-P

aldose; aldehyde group at C_1

fructose 6-P

ketose; keto group at C_2

Shown both in cyclical and linear forms of the sugars.

Figure 2.7: REACTION 3–Second phosphorylation step using ATP.

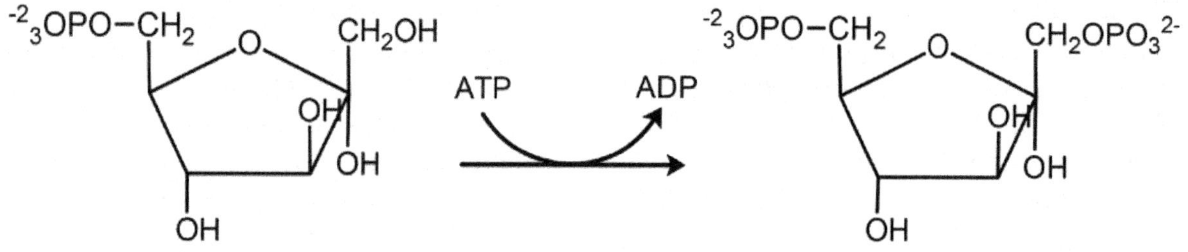

fructose 6-P

fructose 1,6-bisphosphate
(a.k.a. fructose 1,6-BP)

Enzyme: phosphofructokinase (PFK; PFK1)

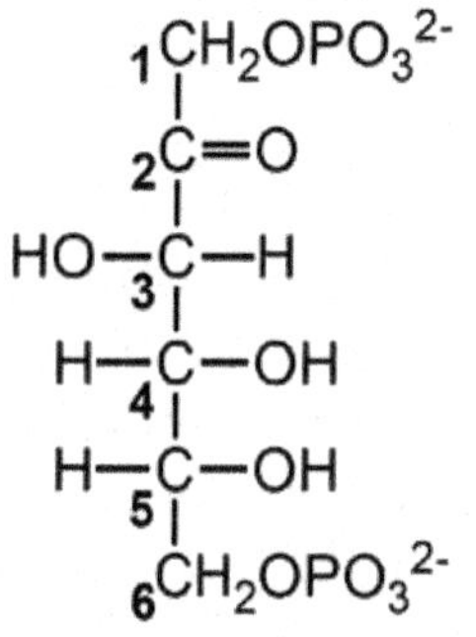

fructose 1,6-BP
(straight chain form)

(Note: Fructose 1,6-BP is shown in both cyclical and linear structures.)

Now that fructose 6-phosphate has a primary alcohol on carbon #1, this hydroxy group can be phosphorylated in reaction #3, as shown in **Figure 2.7**. ATP is the donor of the phosphate group. As expected, the name of the product is fructose 1,6-bisphosphate. The name of the molecule indicates its structure, as long as one knows the structure of fructose. Enzymes that phosphorylate using ATP are called kinases. Kinases are named for the molecule accepting the phosphate from ATP, which is fructose 6-phosphate. One could call the enzyme fructose 6-phosphate kinase. However, the name of the enzyme drops the "6" and puts the "phospho" at the beginning of the enzyme name to call it **phosphofructokinase** (PFK). [Notice the enzyme name is <u>not</u> "bisphosphofructokinase," which would indicate the name for the product of the reaction.] The enzyme is commonly abbreviated as PFK, and to be very specific PFK1 for **phosphofructokinase 1**. There is a phosphofructokinase 2 (PFK2) that is involved in the regulation of this step, which will be discussed later regarding the regulation of glycolysis.

Phosphofructokinase catalyzes another irreversible step of glycolysis. There are four kinase reactions in glycolysis, and three out of the four kinase reactions are irreversible. The ΔG of this reaction is about -5.0 kcal/mol, so there is nothing the cell can do to reverse the reaction. Again, the cleavage of the alcohol phosphate bond on carbon #1 of fructose 1,6-bisphosphate does not have enough energy needed to create a phosphoanhydride bond of ATP for the reverse reaction. This reaction is the "committed step" of glycolysis and it is highly regulated. Once the cell makes fructose 1,6-bisphosphate from PFK1, this molecule will continue on through glycolysis.

Recall that one of the goals of glycolysis is to make ATP. The pathway starts with glucose, which has no phosphates, and the product of the pathway, pyruvate, also has no phosphates. The goal, then, is to take the phosphates that are being put on this molecule and use them to create more ATP. How will the cell achieve a net yield of ATP when it has used two ATP molecules to put on the two phosphate groups, so far? The cell will need to attach more phosphate groups to the molecule that do not require the use of ATP.

Now the cell has phosphorylated the end carbons, as was the goal. The cell is now ready to cut fructose 1,6-bisphosphate in half for reaction #4, forming two 3-carbon molecules, each containing a phosphate group, as shown in **Figure 2.8**. **Figure 2.8** shows fructose 1,6-bisphosphate in its linear form (rather than its normal cyclical form) to indicate how the molecule is divided. This figure, though, does not imply anything regarding the actual enzymatic mechanism. The molecular names of the two products indicate their structures, if one knows two of the key structures shown in **Figure 2.1**: acetone and glycerol. The structure of acetone was the ketone molecule that was also drawn in the oxidation states flow chart (**Figure 1.7**). Glycerol is another simple molecule to draw as it has three carbons with a hydroxy group on each carbon. A carbon makes four bonds, so fill in the remaining carbon bonds with hydrogens to complete the structure of glycerol. If one can draw those two molecules, the rest of the glycolytic intermediates (except for the last reaction) can be drawn based on the names of the structures.

When fructose 1,6-bisphosphate is cut in half, the products of the reaction are two 3-carbon molecules. One of the products is a ketone, dihydroxyacetone phosphate (DHAP), and the other product is an aldehyde, glyceraldehyde 3-phosphate (G3P). For dihydroxyacetone phosphate, first draw acetone but replace one hydrogen on each end carbon with a hydroxy group—i.e. dihydroxyacetone. Since this is a symmetrical molecule, pick one of hydroxy groups and put a phosphate group on it to complete the structure for dihydroxyacetone phosphate. In **Figure 2.8**, the phosphate is put on the end carbon that matches how fructose 1,6-bisphosphate would be drawn cut in half to produce the ketone. It is best to learn the entire name of the molecule, not simply the abbreviation, DHAP. Dihydroxyacetone phosphate, the full name of the molecule, indicates its molecular structure.

Figure 2.8: REACTION 4–Cleavage of fructose 1,6-BP into two 3-carbon phosphorylated molecules

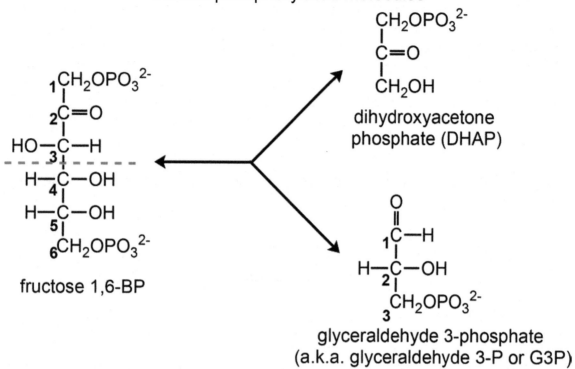

fructose 1,6-BP

dihydroxyacetone phosphate (DHAP)

glyceraldehyde 3-phosphate
(a.k.a. glyceraldehyde 3-P or G3P)

Enzyme: fructose 1,6-bisphosphate aldolase (a.k.a. aldolase)

Glyceraldehyde 3-phosphate is the aldehyde product of this reaction. For this molecule, first draw glycerol, but draw an aldehyde functionality on one of the end carbons (instead of the hydroxy group and hydrogens) forming glyceraldehyde. The aldehyde group is the highest oxidation state on this carbon, which makes this carbon #1. The name of the molecule is glyceraldehyde 3-phosphate, which means the phosphate group is drawn on the hydroxy group of carbon #3—the other end carbon. Now the two products of this reaction have been drawn, dihydroxyacetone phosphate and glyceraldehyde 3-phosphate.

This reaction is very endergonic under standard $\Delta G^{o\prime}$ conditions (about +5.7 kcal/mol), but in the cell the ΔG is only about -0.5 kcal/mole, which makes the reaction readily reversible. The enzyme for reaction #4 is named for a classic organic reaction called an aldol cleavage. An aldol cleavage is a reaction in which a molecule is cleaved to form the products of an aldehyde and a ketone. An aldol condensation, which is the reverse reaction, is a reaction that combines an aldehyde and a ketone to form a larger product. Thus, the enzyme name for this reaction is *fructose 1,6-bisphosphate aldolase*, or more commonly known simply as *aldolase*.

Now consider the two products of reaction #4. Dihydroxyacetone phosphate has a ketone group, which is a functional group that cannot be further oxidized. Glyceraldehyde 3-phosphate, though, has an aldehyde group that can be further oxidized to a carboxylic acid—a goal of catabolic processes. *Therefore, glyceraldehyde 3-phosphate is the molecule that can proceed through the rest of glycolysis.* A keto group, while it cannot be further oxidized to a carboxylic acid, can be isomerized to an aldehyde—and then oxidized to a carboxylic acid. Compare the molecules of dihydroxyacetone phosphate and glyceraldehyde 3-phosphate. Both molecules have the same number of carbons, oxygens, hydrogens, and phosphates. These two molecules are isomers of one another.

Figure 2.9: REACTION 5–Isomerization of DHAP to Glyceraldehyde 3-P

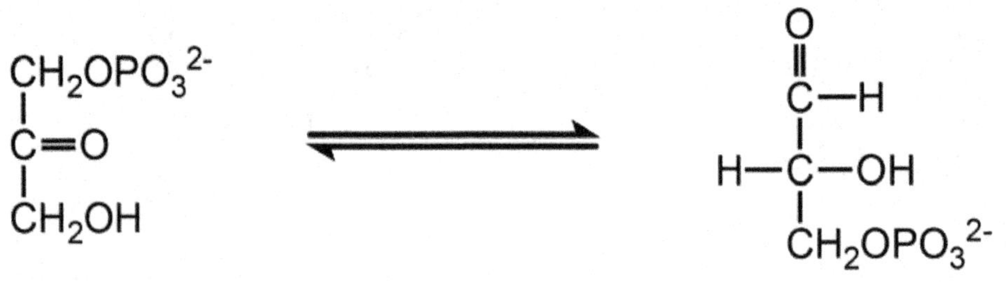

dihydroxyacetone
phosphate (DHAP)

[a ketose]

glyceraldehyde 3-P
(G3P)

[an aldose]

Enzyme: triose phosphate isomerase

Reaction #5, shown in **Figure 2.9**, isomerizes the dihydroxyacetone phosphate (the ketone) to glyceraldehyde 3-phosphate, which are at the same oxidation state. The enzyme that catalyzes this reaction is, therefore, called an isomerase. Again, there are no standard naming conventions for isomerases. These two molecules are, in general terms, 3-carbon phosphorylated sugars—i.e. triose phosphates. Thus, the enzyme name is ***triose phosphate isomerase***. This reaction is rapid and readily reversible. A pool of both molecules is needed to carry out reactions in the cell. At equilibrium there is actually more dihydroxyacetone phosphate than glyceraldehyde 3-phosphate. Remember, though, how metabolism works—maintaining a particular ratio of products to reactants will allow cellular reactions to go in the direction necessary. Keeping the concentration of products low and the concentration of the reactants high will cause the reaction to go in the direction needed. By using the glyceraldehyde 3-phosphate, as soon as it is formed, in the next reaction forces more dihydroxyacetone phosphate to be isomerized to glyceraldehyde 3-phosphate.

At this point, for the purposes of ultimately calculating the maximum yield of ATP from the complete catabolism of a molecule of glucose, there are now two molecules of glyceraldehyde 3-phosphate that will continue through the remainder of glycolysis. The rest of the reactions of glycolysis will then be carried out two times.

Figure 2.10 shows the last five reactions of glycolysis with all the structures. Refer to this figure to review how these last five reactions are carried out in sequence. As the last half of glycolysis is covered, one needs to keep in mind the goals of glycolysis: the pathway is working to get carbons oxidized to carboxylic acids, as well as set up to be good leaving groups as CO_2, and to produce ATP.

Figure 2.10: Glycolysis—the last 5 steps

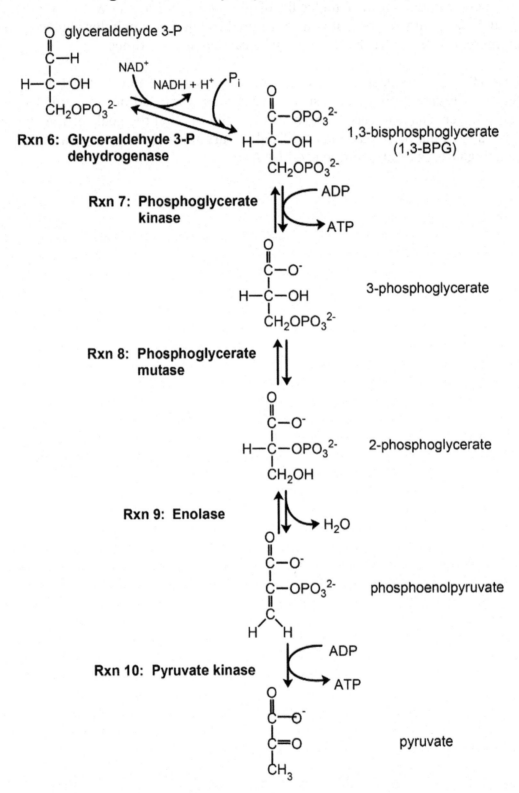

The sequence shown for reaction #6 in **Figure 2.11** is not mechanistically correct. The actual enzyme mechanism does not produce the intermediate shown, which is 3-phosphoglycerate. 3-Phosphoglycerate is an intermediate of glycolysis, but it is not an actual intermediate of reaction #6. The true reaction intermediate is attached to a sulfhydryl group of the enzyme, ultimately forming a thioester. The simplified reaction sequence shown is based on the patterns indicated in the oxidation states flow chart (**Figure 1.7**). In reaction #6, the simplified scheme shows that the enzyme carries out two steps. In the first step, the aldehyde group of glyceraldehyde 3-phosphate will be oxidized to a carboxylic acid. The next step is to add a phosphate group to the carboxylic acid group using inorganic phosphate (P_i), rather than ATP as a donor.

Figure 2.11: REACTION 6–Oxidation/phosphorylation of glyceraldehyde 3-P

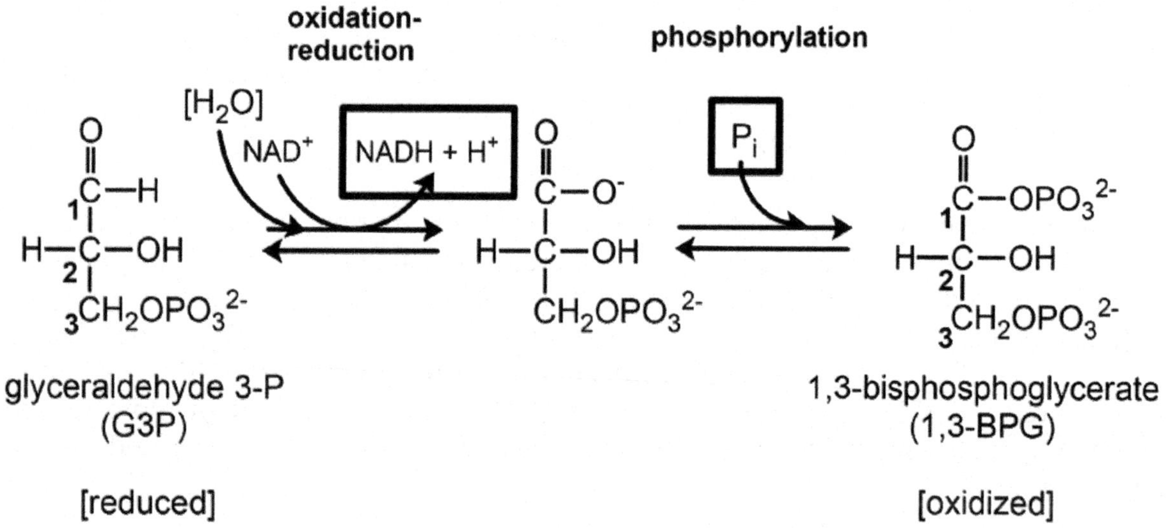

Enzyme: glyceraldehyde 3-phosphate dehydrogenase (GAPDH)

In the first step of reaction #6, the molecule of water needed to go from an aldehyde to a carboxylic acid (as shown in the oxidation states flow chart, **Figure 1.7**) is shown in the figure, though it is not used in the actual reaction mechanism. Recall, though, only part of the water molecule is added, which is why this is an oxidation-reduction reaction and not a hydration reaction. One of the hydrogens is lost from the aldehyde group and one of the hydrogens is lost from the water molecule. Oxidation and reduction reactions are always coupled. As mentioned in the oxidation states chapter, FAD is used when oxidizing an alkane to an alkene. All other oxidations use NAD^+. In this reaction an aldehyde is oxidized to a carboxylic acid, hence NAD^+ is reduced to $NADH + H^+$.

The second step is the phosphorylation of the –OH group (or –O⁻, if deprotonated, as shown in the figure) on the carboxylic acid. However, the cell does not want to use ATP anymore because the goal is to get a net production of ATP. Two ATP were used to put the phosphate groups on the two molecules of glyceraldehyde 3-phosphate created. Inorganic phosphate (P_i, or HPO_4^{2-}) is now used to phosphorylate the carboxylic acid group—not ATP.

The final product of this enzymatic reaction is 1,3-bisphosphoglycerate. The name indicates the structure of the molecule. The –ate ending indicates a deprotonated carboxylic acid group (i.e. carboxylate ion) on the "base structure" of glycerol. Draw glycerol, but draw a deprotonated carboxylic acid group on an end carbon (instead of the –OH group and hydrogens). This would be the molecule "glycerate". A carboxylic acid group is the highest oxidation state, so that carbon becomes carbon #1 of the molecule. The name of the molecule indicates that there are two phosphate groups ("bisphospho"). One of the phosphate groups is on carbon #1, the other is on carbon #3—as shown in **Figure 2.11**. At this point, there are now two molecules of 1,3-bisphosphoglycerate because this reaction will be done two times for the two molecules of glyceraldehyde 3-phosphate. With two molecules of 1,3-bisphosphoglycerate, there are now four phosphate groups that will be used to create four molecules of ATP (for a net yield of two ATP) by the end of the glycolytic pathway—which is not a lot, but often adequate when oxygen is lacking.

For naming the enzyme that carries out these reactions, anytime an enzyme carries out multiple reactions and one of them is a redox reaction using NAD^+ or FAD, the enzyme is always called a *dehydrogenase*. Dehydrogenases are always name for the <u>more reduced</u> molecule, which is glyceraldehyde 3-phosphate for this reaction. This enzyme is then named **glyceraldehyde 3-phosphate dehydrogenase**, which is often abbreviated as GAPDH (pronounced "gap" "D" "H"). The full name, though, indicates the reaction. It is recommended to only use the abbreviation after one has learned the full enzyme name.

This is the only oxidation-reduction step in the entire pathway of glycolysis, and it couples oxidation with phosphorylation. This reaction is readily reversible. What happens to the NADH formed in this reaction (i.e. how the cell regenerates cytosolic NAD^+) is the difference between aerobic and anaerobic glycolysis. The cell must have a pool of cytosolic NAD^+ (the oxidized form) for it to do this reaction.

Another key point is that there are now four phosphate groups to ultimately be removed for the formation of four ATP molecules, two phosphates per molecule of 1,3-bisphosphoglycerate. However, these phosphate groups must be good leaving groups and have enough energy to create a phosphoanhydride bond of ATP that has inherently about -7.3 kcal/mol. [Note that some energy is always lost as heat.] The phosphate group attached to the carboxylic acid group of carbon #1 has a $\Delta G^{o'}$ of about -11.5 kcal/mol, which is more than enough energy to create a bond that has -7.3 kcal/mol. The alcohol phosphate on carbon #3 only has a $\Delta G^{o'}$ of about -3 kcal/mol. The phosphate group on carbon #1 will leave first, and the remaining steps of glycolysis will need to elevate the leaving potential of the phosphate group on carbon #3.

Figure 2.12: REACTION 7–Formation of first ATP

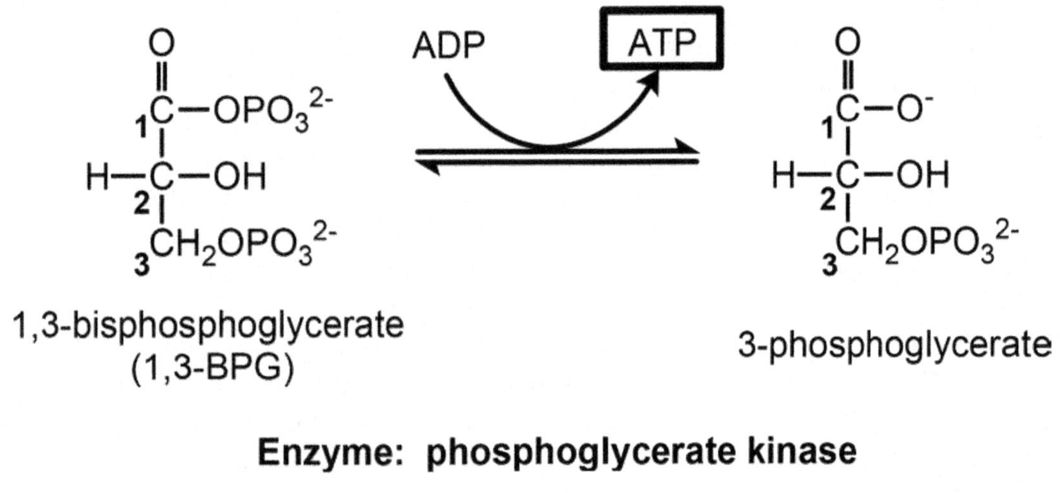

1,3-bisphosphoglycerate
(1,3-BPG)

3-phosphoglycerate

Enzyme: phosphoglycerate kinase

Reaction #7, as shown in **Figure 2.12**, produces the formation of the first ATP. This reaction is where the cell "breaks even" in its yield of ATP from glycolysis. Two molecules of 1,3-bisphosphoglycerate go through this reaction to produce two ATP, but the pathway used 2 ATP in the first half. The phosphate group from carbon #1 of 1,3-bisphosphoglycerate was transferred to ADP to make ATP forming the product 3-phosphoglycerate, whose the name indicates its structure. The -ate indicates that the molecule has a deprotonated carboxylic acid group on the "base molecule" glycerol—forming "glycerate." The carboxylic acid carbon is carbon #1, as the highest oxidation state. Thus, the phosphate group is on the hydroxy group of the other end carbon, carbon #3.

This reaction is carried out by a kinase, though it may not look like it because a kinase is an enzyme that transfers a phosphate from ATP to an acceptor. This reaction is producing ATP. Reaction #7 is termed a "substrate level phosphorylation" reaction because it transfers a high energy phosphate leaving group from an organic molecule to ADP to make ATP. In contrast, oxidative phosphorylation is carried out by the electron transport chain. Oxidative phosphorylation couples the energy created from a proton gradient produced by the movement of electrons to the phosphorylation of ADP to make ATP. There are not many enzymes that can create a phosphoanhydride bond of ATP via a substrate level phosphorylation reaction. The enzyme that catalyzes reaction #7, and the enzyme that catalyzes reaction #10, are kinases. These two kinases are named for the reverse reactions. Naming the enzyme for the reverse reaction is the correct way to name the kinase—as if ATP is donating a phosphate group to an acceptor molecule, 3-phosphoglycerate. The enzyme is called ***phosphoglycerate kinase***, as the enzyme name does not include the "3." The reaction catalyzed by phosphoglycerate kinase is the only kinase reaction, of the four kinase reactions in glycolysis, that is actually reversible.

Now consider what needs to happen in the last three steps of glycolysis—reactions 8, 9, and 10, which includes application of concepts covered in the oxidation states chapter. At this point in glycolysis, two of the six original carbons of a glucose molecule are now at the level of a carboxylic acid (i.e. two molecules of 3-phosphoglycerate)—one of the goals of catabolic processes. Carboxylic acid groups are stable, though, and are not good leaving groups. In biological systems, a keto group must be placed alpha or beta to the carboxylic acid carbon to make the carboxylic acid group a good leaving group. However, 3-phosphoglycerate is a three-carbon molecule, and a keto group is a carbonyl group attached to two other carbons. Therefore, the only place to put a keto group is on carbon #2 of the molecule, creating an alpha-keto acid. Decarboxylation of an alpha-keto acid is "harder," but it can be done. The decarboxylation of pyruvate, an alpha-keto acid, to form CO_2 does not occur in glycolysis. Two molecules of pyruvate are formed at the end of glycolysis, so all six carbons of the original glucose molecule are still in the cell. Also, the final product, pyruvate, does not have any phosphate groups. Another goal is to make that phosphate group on 3-phosphoglycerate a good enough leaving group that it can be used to phosphorylate ADP to make ATP. Thus, the two goals that must be accomplished by reactions 8, 9, and 10 are to elevate the leaving potential of the phosphate group and create a keto group on carbon #2.

Figure 2.13: REACTION 8–Rearrangement of phosphate group

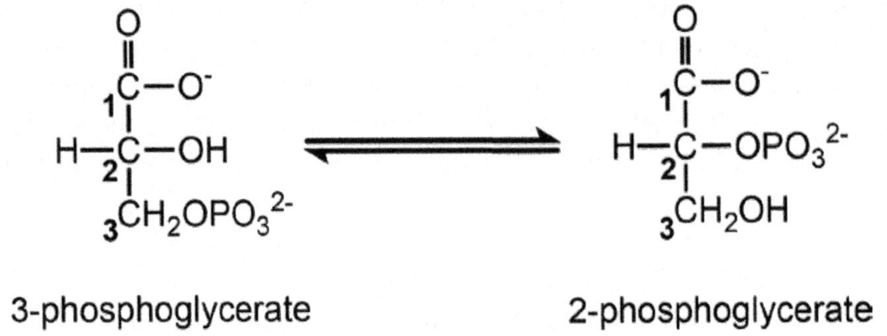

3-phosphoglycerate   2-phosphoglycerate

Enzyme: phosphoglycerate mutase

In reaction #8, shown in **Figure 2.13**, the first step towards accomplishing the two goals is to move the phosphate group from the hydroxy group of carbon #3 to the hydroxy group of carbon #2. The names indicate the structures: 3-phosphoglycerate and 2-phosphoglycerate. Drawing glycerate has already been described; now just draw the phosphate group on the hydroxy group of carbon #2. This is an isomerization reaction and is readily reversible. The number of carbons, hydrogens, oxygens, and phosphates are the same on both molecules, just arranged differently. One could call the enzyme for this reaction an isomerase, but this reaction specifically moved a functional group (i.e. a phosphate group). Enzymes that catalyze intramolecular shifts of functional groups on a molecule (i.e. phosphate groups, amino groups, etc.) are a special class of isomerases called *mutases*. Therefore the name of this enzyme drops the numbers from the molecule names ("2" and "3") to be called *phosphoglycerate mutase*.

It does not seem like this reaction accomplished much because that phosphate group is still in alcohol phosphate group, which a poor leaving group. However, it is the phosphate group that needs to leave and a keto group needs to be created on carbon #2. When the phosphate group leaves from carbon #2, a keto group will be created on carbon #2. That is why the phosphate group is moved to carbon #2. First the phosphate group is moved, and then a reaction is done to elevate its leaving potential.

Figure 2.14: REACTION 9–Formation of an enol phosphate

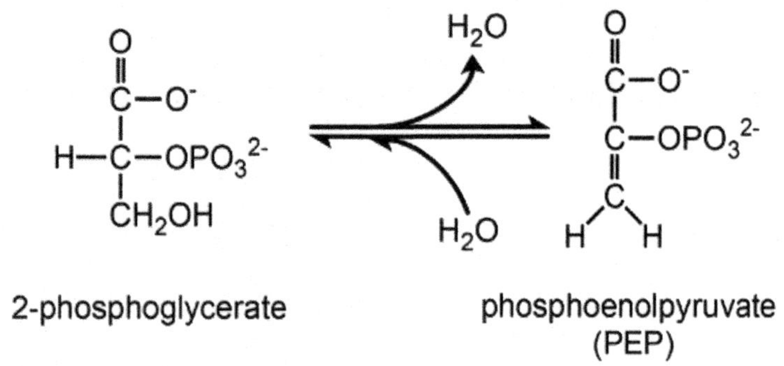

2-phosphoglycerate

phosphoenolpyruvate
(PEP)

Enzyme: enolase

Reaction #9, shown in **Figure 2.14**, forms an enol group, specifically an enol phosphate. This is a dehydration reaction, which is a loss of water from the molecule (i.e. the hydrogen from carbon #2 and the hydroxy group from carbon #3). As shown in the oxidation states basic recipe (**Figure 1.7**), dehydration of a molecule yields a molecule with a double bond (an alkene). This dehydration reaction is reversible.

The dehydration of 2-phosphoglycerate yields phosphoenolpyruvate (PEP), a product that has a double bond between carbons #2 and #3. The name of the product, phosphoenolpyruvate, does not explicitly indicate its structure. One needs to know the structure of the 3-carbon molecule pyruvate, formed in reaction #10, to draw the structure based on its name. Phosphoenolpyruvate is three carbons, and the name indicates it has a deprotonated carboxylic acid group (i.e. the "-ate" ending) and an enol phosphate. The "ene" part of "enol" indicates the double bond (i.e. alkene) functional group. The "-ol" of "enol" indicates an alcohol group (hydroxy group), which is still on carbon #2 because the hydroxy group was removed from carbon #3 in this reaction. The phosphate is also still on the hydroxy group of carbon #2, as it was for the substrate 2-phosphoglycerate—forming the "enol phosphate."

Most enzymes that carry out dehydration reactions are called dehydratases and are named for the molecule that loses the water molecule. Most enzymes that carry out hydration reactions are called hydratases and are named after the molecule that gains the water molecule. However, many dehydration and hydration reactions are reversible, so some enzymes names for these types of reactions do not follow the naming rules. The enzyme name for this reaction is an "exception" to the naming rules. The enzyme that catalyzes reaction #9 is simply called *enolase*, for the enol functional group it creates on phosphoenolpyruvate.

The purpose of this dehydration reaction to form an enol phosphate markedly elevates the leaving group potential of the phosphate group. The $\Delta G^{o\prime}$ of the enol phosphate bond is now about -15 kcal/mol, which is more than enough to make a phosphoanhydride bond of ATP. Now this phosphate group can be used to phosphorylate ADP to make ATP. Also, when the phosphate group leaves from carbon #2, a keto group will be formed on that carbon.

Figure 2.15: REACTION 10–Formation of pyruvate and second ATP

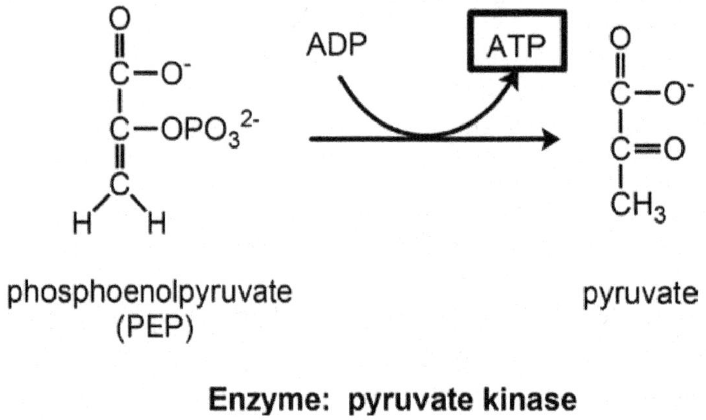

phosphoenolpyruvate
(PEP)

pyruvate

Enzyme: pyruvate kinase

Figure 2.15 shows reaction #10, the last reaction of glycolysis (at least for aerobic glycolysis). This reaction provides the net yield of two ATP for the pathway in the formation of two molecules of pyruvate. In this reaction, the phosphate group on carbon #2 of phosphoenolpyruvate is transferred to ADP to make ATP, resulting in the formation of pyruvate. This reaction is also a substrate level phosphorylation reaction.

The name "pyruvate" does not indicate much about its structure. The –ate ending indicates there is a deprotonated carboxylic acid group (which must be on an end carbon that becomes carbon #1), but this is a structure one must know (like glucose and fructose). Pyruvate is a three carbon alpha-keto acid. Since it is three carbons, the keto group must be on the middle carbon. Therefore draw the keto group on carbon 2, and now draw a methyl group for carbon 3.

As explained for the kinase reaction #6. This enzyme is also going to be called a kinase, but it is named for the reverse reaction. However, this reaction is irreversible. It does not actually go "in reverse." Kinases, though, are always named as if ATP is donating a phosphate group to an acceptor molecule, pyruvate in this case. Therefore this enzyme is called **pyruvate kinase** (<u>not</u> phosphoenolpyruvate kinase).

This reaction is, as mentioned, irreversible with a ΔG of about -5.5 kcal/mol, and it is regulated. Of the four steps in glycolysis that use kinases, three of them are irreversible. These three irreversible steps are the regulated steps of glycolysis.

In this last step of glycolysis, an alpha-keto acid has been formed. There is no loss of carbons in glycolysis, but the two carboxylic acid groups (i.e. two molecules of pyruvate) have been set up as good leaving groups because of the keto group on the alpha carbon of pyruvate. This catabolic pathway has also provided a net yield of 2 ATP. The fate of pyruvate is going to depend on whether molecular oxygen is available, whether pyruvate needs to be further catabolized, or whether certain amino acids are needed. Recall that pyruvate can be converted to alanine easily through a transaminase reaction.

REGULATION OF GLYCOLYSIS

Another key question one should strive to understand about any metabolic pathway is: When? When (i.e. under what conditions) is this pathway activated ("on") or inhibited ("off")? With which other pathways does the cell run the pathway simultaneously or in sequence? Which pathways cannot be "on" simultaneously in the same cell (i.e. reciprocal pathways like glycolysis and gluconeogenesis)? The ability to answer the question "When?" helps one achieve understanding of how metabolic pathways are integrated. Two "basic concepts" of metabolic pathway regulation will be stressed when covering a given metabolic pathway in this text:

> (1) How does the "energy state" of the cell, meaning the ratio of cellular concentrations of ATP to ADP (or AMP), affect the activation or inhibition of the pathway?
> (2) When two enzymes that use the same reactants (i.e. substrates and/or products) are in the same cellular compartment how does the cell regulate which enzyme is active versus inhibited?

Therefore, before discussing the fates of the products of glycolysis, a review of some of the important regulators of glycolysis are presented. Regulation of metabolic pathways is very complex, and includes levels of regulation from the expression of the genes encoding the enzymes, the activities of the expressed enzymes, the accessibility of the substrates and products, as well as the degradation of the enzymes. The glycolytic pathway will be used to present a brief insight into this complexity, but only at the level of activity of the enzymes.

There are three irreversible kinase reactions in glycolysis catalyzed by hexokinase, phosphofructokinase 1 (PFK1), and pyruvate kinase. These three reactions have to be bypassed in the reciprocal pathway of gluconeogenesis, which is the *de novo* synthesis of a molecule of glucose from two molecules of pyruvate. The reactions catalyzed by hexokinase and PFK1 are bypassed in gluconeogenesis using enzymes called phosphatases. A phosphatase is an enzyme that clips a phosphate group off of a molecule and releases it as inorganic phosphate (P_i). For the hexokinase reaction, glucose 6-phosphatase (named for the molecule which loses the phosphate group) is the enzyme that catalyzes the reverse reaction in gluconeogenesis. Only two organs in your body have that enzyme, the liver and kidneys, because they are responsible for maintaining the blood glucose supply. For the phosphofructokinase 1 (PFK1) reaction, *fructose 1,6-bisphosphatase* (FBP1) catalyzes the reverse reaction in gluconeogenesis (shown in **Figure 2.16**; note the full name of FBP1 is written in the lower right corner of the figure). Fructose 1,6-bisphosphatase is also named for the molecule that loses the phosphate group. In gluconeogenesis, bypassing the pyruvate kinase reaction of glycolysis requires two enzymes and a transporter across the inner mitochondrial membrane. These gluconeogenic enzymes are pyruvate carboxylase and phosphoenolpyruvate carboxykinase (PEPCK). Glycolysis and gluconeogenesis cannot be active ("on") simultaneously in the same cell because it would create a "futile cycle," in which glucose is broken down by glycolysis only to be re-synthesized by gluconeogenesis. Running these pathways simultaneously in the same cell would yield no net energy and no chemical or biological work would be done.

Hexokinase is the first regulated step of glycolysis. Recall that hexokinase catalyzes reaction #1, the phosphorylation of glucose by ATP to form glucose 6-phosphate and ADP. Glucose 6-phosphate is an allosteric inhibitor of hexokinase. There is a separate binding site on the enzyme hexokinase for glucose 6-phosphate. As glucose 6-phosphate builds up in a cell, glucose 6-phosphate binds to this allosteric site and inhibits this enzyme. This inhibition helps control glucose uptake into the cell. Recall that glucokinase, the liver isozyme, is not inhibited by glucose 6-phosphate. The hexokinase reaction is not the key regulated step because glucose 6-phosphate does not have to go through glycolysis.

The reaction catalyzed by phosphofructokinase 1 (PFK1) is the committed step of glycolysis and the primary regulatory control point of the pathway. PFK1 catalyzes the phosphorylation of fructose 6-phosphate by ATP to form fructose 1,6-bisphosphate and ADP, as shown in **Figure 2.16**. Phosphofructokinase 1 has several regulatory sites on the enzyme for the binding of several allosteric activators and inhibitors. Allosteric activators of PFK1 include fructose <u>2</u>,6-bisphosphate (which will be covered in detail), ADP, and AMP. Allosteric inhibitors of PFK1 include ATP and citrate. Citrate is a TCA cycle intermediate, but is transported into the cytosol for fatty acid synthesis (as will be covered in lipid metabolism). Citrate, then, serves to coordinate certain aspects of carbohydrate and lipid metabolism.

Figure 2.16: Reciprocal regulation of GLYCOLYSIS and GLUCONEOGENESIS via fructose 2,6-bisphosphate (fructose 2,6-BP).

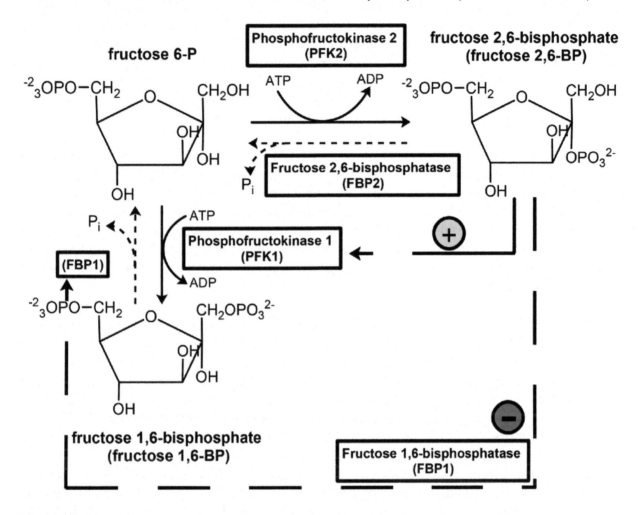

Figure 2.16 notes:

1. Fructose 2,6-bisphosphate is a potent **activator** of PFK1 <u>AND</u> a potent **inhibitor** of FBP1, ensuring that glycolysis and gluconeogenesis are **not** on at the same time in the same cell.

2. PFK2 and FBP2 are in one bifunctional enzyme complex. When one is on, the other one is off.

3. **FBP2** is the enzyme that is <u>hormonally</u> controlled. Glucagon (i.e. low blood sugar) activates FBP2, thus PFK2 is off. Insulin (i.e. high blood sugar) inhibits FBP2, thus PFK2 is now on.

4. <u>**HINT**</u>: When the **kinases are on** (PFK1 and PFK2), **glycolysis** is active in the cell. When the <u>bisphosphatases are on</u> (FBP1 and FBP2), <u>gluconeogenesis</u> is active in the cell.

The "energy state" of the cell controls PFK1 and the flux of glucose through glycolysis. As a purpose of the catabolism of glucose is to produce ATP, the major chemical form of energy for the cell, high cellular concentrations of ATP inhibit PFK1 as ATP binds to the allosteric sites on the enzyme. Glycolysis is inhibited, as one would expect. As ATP is consumed by cellular reactions, the concentrations of ADP and AMP rise in the cell. ADP and AMP, then, serve as activators of PFK1 and increase the flux of glucose through glycolysis to produce more ATP. High levels of ATP in a cell generally result in the inhibition of catabolic processes, whose purposes include the generation of reducing power leading to ATP production by the electron transport chain.

Pyruvate kinase, which catalyzes reaction #10 of glycolysis, is the third regulated step of glycolysis. Pyruvate kinase catalyzes the formation of ATP and pyruvate from phosphoenolpyruvate (PEP) and ADP. Fructose 1,6-bisphosphate is an allosteric activator of pyruvate kinase. This activation by an intermediate formed earlier in the pathway is termed "feed-forward" activation. As this is the glycolytic step that results in the net yield of ATP, it is important the pyruvate kinase is already active and "ready' to convert PEP to pyruvate to form ATP. High cellular concentrations of ATP, as one would expect, also inhibit pyruvate kinase.

There are also isozymes of pyruvate kinase, the liver isozyme (L form) and the muscle isozyme (M form). The liver isozyme of pyruvate kinase is regulated by reversible phosphorylation of the enzyme, which is controlled by hormones. Insulin is the hormone that indicates the blood glucose level is "high" and stimulates the tissues that are targeted by insulin to take up glucose, as necessary, for their needs. Glucagon indicates the blood glucose level is low. The ratio of insulin to glucagon in the blood is important, more so than the individual concentrations of each hormone.

The liver is a target tissue of both insulin and glucagon. The liver must remove excess glucose from the blood, and it (along with the kidneys) is responsible for maintaining the blood glucose levels. The liver and kidneys are the only organs that have the enzyme glucose 6-phosphatase that allows glucose to be released back into the blood. Glucagon would lead to stimulation of gluconeogenesis in the liver; while insulin stimulates glycolysis.

Now consider when pyruvate kinase, a glycolytic enzyme, should be activated or inhibited. When gluconeogenesis is occurring in a liver cell, pyruvate kinase would need to be "off" or inhibited. Pyruvate kinase needs to be "on" or active during glycolysis. **Insulin** ultimately leads to the **dephosphorylation** of the L isozyme of pyruvate kinase to **activate** it because insulin activates the pathway of glycolysis. *Glucagon* ultimately leads to the *phosphorylation* of the L isozyme of pyruvate kinase to *inhibit* it because glucagon leads to the activation of gluconeogenesis.

The next basic concept of regulation that will be covered is the reciprocal control of two enzymes, simultaneously, by one effector molecule. In this case, phosphofructokinase 1 (PFK1) of glycolysis and fructose 1,6-bisphosphatase (FBP1) of gluconeogenesis both utilize fructose 6-phosphate and fructose 1,6-bisphosphate (see **Figure 2.16**, the reverse reactions drawn vertically on the left side of the figure). In *glycolysis*, phosphofructokinase 1 (PFK1) catalyzes the reaction of fructose 6-phosphate + ATP to from fructose 1,6-bisphospate + ADP. In *gluconeogenesis*, fructose 1,6-bisphosphatase (FBP1) catalyzes the reaction of fructose 1,6-bisphosphate to form fructose 6-phosphate + P_i. Glycolysis and gluconeogenesis are reciprocal pathways, and therefore are not on in the same cell at the same time, as previously discussed.

How does the cell regulate which direction the reaction needs to go? Fructose <u>2</u>,6-bisphosphate is a single effector molecule that controls both enzymes, PFK1 and FBP1—because they cannot both be on at the same time in the same cell. Fructose 2,6-bisphosphate, as its name implies, indicates it has phosphate groups on the hydroxy groups of carbons #2 and #6 of fructose (not carbons #1 and #6, as on fructose 1,6-bisphosphate). The structure of the effector molecule, fructose 2,6-bisphosphate is shown in **Figure 2.16** at the upper right of the figure. This production of this effector molecule is used solely for regulating PFK1 and FBP1. Fructose 2,6-bisphosphate is not an intermediate for other reactions of glycolysis or gluconeogenesis. Both PFK1 and FBP1 have allosteric binding sites for the molecule fructose 2,6-bisphosphate (i.e. not the catalytic sites of either enzyme). The purpose of fructose 2,6-bisphosphate is to bind to both of these enzymes to turn one of them on, and the other one off. To understand which one of them is "on" in the presence of fructose 2,6-bisphosphate, one needs to understand how this effector molecule is made and when the cell the is able to make it.

The synthesis of fructose 2,6-bisphosphate is shown in **Figure 2.16**, as the two horizontal reactions at the top of the figure from left to right. Fructose 2,6-bisphosphate is made from fructose 6-phosphate. The phosphate group that is attached to the hydroxy group of carbon #2 comes from ATP. Enzymes that phosphorylate molecules using ATP are called kinases and are named after the acceptor of the phosphate—in this case, fructose 6-phosphate. Hence this enzyme is also call phosphofructokinase, but now we call it phosphofructokinase 2 (PFK2). So now we have PFK1 and PFK2.

This effector molecule must also be able to be removed from the cell, which will reverse which enzyme (i.e. PFK1 and FBP1) is active and which enzyme is inhibited. The formation of fructose 2,6-bisphosphate by PFK2 is also an irreversible reaction (just like the PFK1 catalyzed reaction). Therefore a different enzyme is needed to remove the phosphate group from fructose 2,6-bisphosphate to re-form fructose 6-phosphate and inorganic phosphate (P_i). The enzyme that catalyzes the reverse reaction is a phosphatase named for the molecule that loses the phosphate group—*fructose 2,6-bisphosphatase* (FBP2). The enzyme names make sense. For PFK<u>1</u> and FBP<u>1</u> the enzymes are either adding a phosphate group or removing a phosphate group from <u>carbon #1</u> of a fructose derivative, respectively. For PFK<u>2</u> and FBP<u>2</u> the enzymes are either adding a phosphate group or removing a phosphate group from <u>carbon #2</u> of a fructose derivative, respectively. PFK2 and FBP2 actually exist together as an enzyme complex, in which one of them is hormonally controlled. Fructose 2,6-bisphosphatase (FBP2) is hormonally controlled by reversible phosphorylation.

Now consider under what conditions should phosphofructokinase 1 (PFK1) and fructose 1,6-bisphosphatase (FBP1) be on or off? Fructose 2,6-bisphosphate is an effector molecule made from fructose 6-phosphate by a kinase that requires ATP. This effector molecule can only be made when there is plenty of glucose available because some of the fructose 6-phosphate will be diverted to make it. Therefore, the effector molecule fructose 2,6-bisphosphate should turn on phosphofructokinase 1 (PFK1) because the cell can do glycolysis when plenty of glucose is available. Fructose 2,6-bisphosphate binds to an allosteric site on PFK1 to activate it, and it binds to an allosteric site on fructose 1,6-bisphosphatase (FBP1) to inhibit it (shown in **Figure 2.16** by the dotted lines with the (+) and (-) signs indicating activation or inhibition of the respective enzymes). *Insulin*, as a hormonal control of fructose 2,6-bisphosphatase (FBP2), *dephosphorylates* the FBP2 to *inactive* it; resulting in the <u>activation of PFK2</u> to make the effector molecule fructose 2,6-bisphosphate.

When the cell needs to carry out *de novo* synthesis of glucose via gluconeogenesis, then all molecules that can become a glucose molecule need to be converted to glucose. Under these conditions, the effector fructose 2,6-bisphosphate molecules need to be converted back to fructose 6-phosphate molecules via fructose 2,6-bisphosphatase (FBP2). The fructose 6-phosphate will then continue through gluconeogenesis back to form glucose molecules. As fructose 2,6-bisphosphate is removed, phosphofructokinase 1 (PFK1) of glycolysis is inhibited and fructose 1,6-bisphosphatse (FBP1) of gluconeogenesis is activated. Glucagon is the hormone that signals low blood glucose levels, and the liver responds by releasing glucose into the blood. *Glucagon*, therefore, *phosphorylates* FBP2 to turn *activate* it, and <u>PFK2 will be inhibited</u> under these conditions.

This complex reciprocal regulatory concept by fructose 2,6-bisphosphatase can be simplified into two "rules":

1. When the kinases are on (meaning PFK1 and PFK2), the cell is doing glycolysis; and FBP1 and FBP2 are off under these conditions.
2. When the bisphosphatases are on (meaning FBP1 and FBP2), the cell is doing gluconeogenesis; and the kinases, PFK1 and PFK2 are off.

The key point is that when the cell has two enzymes in the same compartment using the same intermediates, the regulation of both enzymes is important to directing the flux of intermediates into the necessary pathway.

METABOLIC FATES OF THE PRODUCTS OF GLYCOLYSIS

What happens to the products made in glycolysis, ATP, NADH and pyruvate? ATP is the primary form of chemical energy for cells. The hydrolysis of ATP is used to drive many endergonic reactions and processes, and is used in synthetic (anabolic) pathways, which generally require energy input to create larger molecules. One of the main purposes of glycolysis is that this catabolic pathway yields ATP directly, without the need of the electron transport chain.

Glycolysis also produces NADH and pyruvate. The fate of both of these molecules will depend on the availability of molecular oxygen (O_2). Molecular oxygen, though, is not used in any of the reactions of glycolysis. Why, then, would oxygen availability control the fate of products of glycolysis? Molecular oxygen is the final electron acceptor of the electron transport chain, located in the inner mitochondrial membrane. The reducing power of NADH and $FADH_2$, produced by catabolic pathways, are the electron donors to the electron transport chain. The movement of these electrons through the complexes of the ETC, ending up on O_2 to reduce it to water, produces a proton gradient. The proton gradient is coupled to the phosphorylation of ADP by P_i to form ATP. The electron transport chain is the major pathway for the production of ATP from nutrient catabolism, and requires reducing power from catabolic pathways and oxygen.

Recall that the pathway of glycolysis is in the cytosol. The NADH produced by the glyceraldehyde 3-P dehydrogenase reaction is in the cytosol. The "pools" of cytosolic NAD^+/NADH and mitochondrial NAD^+/NADH are kept separate. The entire molecule of NAD^+ or NADH is not allowed to cross the inner mitochondrial membrane. Think of it in the following terms: if the cell sends the whole NADH molecule into the mitochondria to give its electrons to the ETC, then the NAD^+ formed in the matrix will not come back out to the cytosol because there are many more reactions in the mitochondria that use NAD^+ and NADH. However, it is not the entire NADH molecule that needs to go the electron transport chain, just the electrons that it is carrying. The movement of the electrons on the cytosolic NADH formed in glycolysis will be transported to the electron transport chain using "shuttles". There are two shuttles, which will be discussed, the malate-aspartate shuttle and the glycerol phosphate shuttle. The shuttles only work under **aerobic** conditions because that is when the electron transport chain is working and can use the electrons from the cytosolic NADH molecule. Under aerobic conditions, the shuttles are how cytosolic NAD^+ is re-generated for the glyceraldehyde 3-P dehydrogenase step to continue.

Under aerobic conditions, pyruvate can also be transported into the mitochondrial matrix to continue the catabolism of pyruvate via the pyruvate dehydrogenase (PDH) complex and the tricarboxylic acid (TCA) cycle. The continued catabolism of pyruvate in the matrix will yield carbon dioxide (CO_2), reducing power (NADH and $FADH_2$), and ultimately more ATP via the electron transport chain (ETC).

Now consider what happens under anaerobic conditions, when there is not enough molecular oxygen to allow the electron transport chain to continue working. If the electron transport chain is inhibited, then the PDH complex and the TCA cycle in the mitochondria are also inhibited because the reducing power produced cannot go the ETC. If the cell still needs to generate ATP under these conditions, glycolysis becomes the only catabolic process producing a net yield of ATP directly (via substrate level phosphorylation reactions). The ten reactions of glycolysis still produce NADH (at the glyceraldehyde 3-P dehydrogenase step) and pyruvate (as the product of the pyruvate kinase step). The electron transport chain is not operating, so the electrons from the cytosolic NADH cannot be shuttled to the ETC, and pyruvate cannot be further catabolized by the PDH complex and the TCA cycle.

There is still the problem of re-generating cytosolic NAD^+. If glycolysis becomes the cell's only catabolic pathway generating ATP, a pool of cytosolic NAD^+ for the glyceraldehyde 3-phosphate dehydrogenase step still needs to be maintained. This is the importance of the location of glycolysis in the cytosol, not in the mitochondria. If glycolysis was in the mitochondria, it would depend on the electron transport chain to regenerate its supply of NAD^+, as most other catabolic process do.

Figure 2.17: REACTION 11–Formation of lactate from pyruvate.

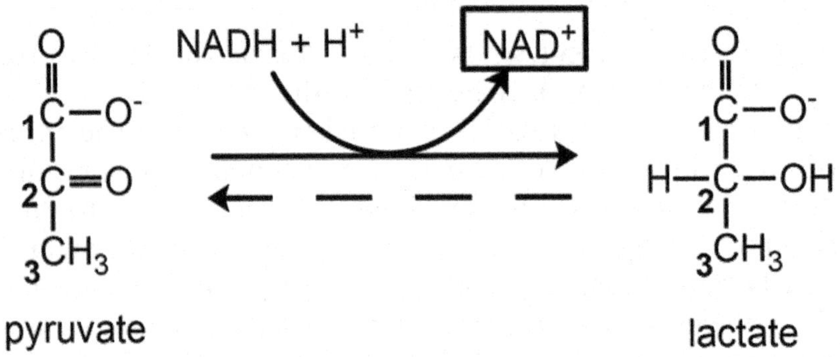

Enzyme: lactate dehydrogenase
(Anaerobic conditions only—anaerobic glycolysis.)

To re-generate cytosolic NAD^+ under anaerobic conditions, pyruvate stays in the cytosol, as it also cannot be transported into the mitochondria. Recall that pyruvate has a keto group on carbon #2. Under anaerobic conditions glycolysis carries out an eleventh reaction (shown in **Figure 2.17**), in which the keto group of pyruvate is reduced to form a secondary alcohol, producing the molecule lactate. This is a reduction reaction. If a molecule is reduced, a molecule must be oxidizes. Normally to go "up" the oxidation states flow chart (**Figure 1.7**), the cell should use $NADPH + H^+$ and oxidize it to $NADP^+$. However, the sole purpose of this reaction is to regenerate cytosolic NAD^+ for glycolysis to continue. This reaction does, indeed, use **$NADH + H^+$** and oxidizes it to **NAD^+**. Enzymes that carry out redox reactions that use and $NAD^+/NADH$ or $FAD/FADH_2$ are called *dehydrogenases*. Dehydrogenases are named for the more reduced molecule, which is lactate. Thus, the enzyme name is ***lactate dehydrogenase***. Now cytosolic NAD^+ is regenerated for the glyceraldehyde 3-P dehydrogenase reaction, so glycolysis can continue to make ATP under anaerobic conditions, when the ETC is not working.

The lactate dehydrogenase reaction is a reversible reaction. The liver, however, is the primary organ that can form pyruvate from lactate. All other tissues that generate lactate, especially muscle and red blood cells, will send the lactate back to the liver. Recall, as discussed previously, mature red blood cells do not have mitochondria and can only generate ATP by anaerobic glycolysis. The liver uses the lactate is a source of pyruvate for the pathway of gluconeogenesis to synthesize glucose, which released into the blood and sent as a energy source for muscle and red blood cells. This process is called the **Cori Cycle**.

SHUTTLES FOR TRANSPORT OF CYTOSOLIC NADH ELECTRONS

(Aerobic glycolysis)
Under aerobic conditions glycolysis has 10 reactions and uses one of the shuttles to regenerate its cytosolic pool of NAD^+; while under anaerobic conditions, glycolysis consists of 11 reactions. The **malate-aspartate shuttle** and the **glycerol phosphate shuttle** are the two shuttles used by various tissues of the body.

(What?) The malate-aspartate shuttle and the glycerol phosphate shuttle, under aerobic conditions, shuttle the **2 electrons** from cytosolic NADH into the mitochondria and generate either a mitochondrial NADH (for the malate-aspartate shuttle) or a mitochondrial $FADH_2$ (for the glycerol phosphate shuttle). **(Why?)** These shuttles have now regenerated cytosolic NAD^+ for glycolysis to continue, and the mitochondrial NADH or $FADH_2$ deliver these 2 electrons to the electron transport chain, which can be used to make ATP. These shuttles only transport the 2 *electrons* from cytosolic NADH, not the whole molecule of NADH.

(Where?) In the cell, these shuttles involve enzymatic reactions in both the cytosol and the mitochondria. The malate-aspartate shuttle is used by all tissues, and the heart and liver use it exclusively as it is the more energy-efficient shuttle. The glycerol phosphate shuttle is used by most tissues as a secondary mechanism for transporting electrons to the mitochondria.

(How?) The malate-aspartate shuttle is shown in **Figure 2.18**. As the purpose of the shuttle is to move electrons, the shuttle involves oxidation-reductions. In **Figure 2.18**, begin with the molecules of NADH and oxaloacetate in the cytosol (lower left of the figure). Cytosolic malate dehydrogenase reduces oxaloacetate to malate with the simultaneous oxidation of NADH + H^+ back to NAD^+. The first goal of the shuttle has now been met—the regeneration of cytosolic NAD^+ for glycolysis to continue. Malate crosses into the mitochondrial matrix where mitochondrial malate dehydrogenase oxidizes the malate to oxaloacetate and forms a mitochondrial molecule of NADH. [Note that this enzymatic reaction will be covered in more detail in the TCA cycle.] This mitochondrial NADH can deliver its two electrons to the electron transport chain for the ultimate synthesis of ATP, the second goal of the shuttle.

There must be a pool of cytosolic oxaloacetate for this shuttle to operate, but oxaloacetate cannot cross the inner mitochondrial membrane. Therefore, a series of transamination reactions occur to regenerate the cytosolic pool of oxaloacetate. The relationship between alpha-keto acids and alpha-amino acids and their inter-conversion by transamination reactions was covered in chapter 1 (see **Figure 1.5**). In the mitochondria, the alpha-amino group of glutamate is removed by the mitochondrial aspartate aminotransferase (AST) forming α-ketoglutarate. The mitochondrial AST then transfers the amino group to oxaloacetate to form the amino acid aspartate. The aspartate is transported to the cytosol where a cytosolic AST reverses the transamination reaction to generate cytosolic oxaloacetate.

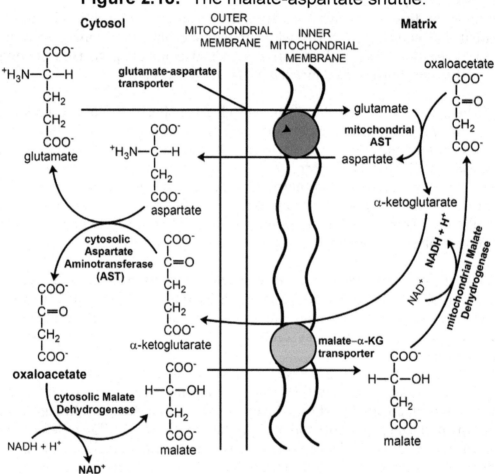

Figure 2.18: The malate-aspartate shuttle.

[NOTE: Start with **oxaloacetate** in the cytosol.]

The malate-aspartate shuttle is readily <u>reversible</u> (unlike the glycerol phosphate shuttle). Thus NADH electrons can only be transferred to the mitochondria when the NADH/NAD⁺ ratio is higher in the cytosol than in the mitochondria. Gluconeogenesis, in fact, depends on this shuttle running in reverse to move the mitochondrial oxaloacetate formed by pyruvate carboxylase to the cytosol by reducing it to malate.

The glycerol phosphate shuttle is shown in **Figure 2.19**. In this shuttle, cytosolic dihydroxyacetone phosphate is needed. Recall that dihydroxyacetone phosphate is the glycolytic intermediate formed by reaction #4 of glycolysis when fructose 1,6-bisphosphate is cut in half. In the first reaction of this shuttle, cytosolic *glycerol phosphate dehydrogenase* (a.k.a. *glycerophosphate dehydrogenase*) reduces the keto group of dihydroxyacetone to form glycerol phosphate (whose name indicates its structure) with the simultaneous oxidation of cytosolic NADH + H$^+$ back to NAD$^+$. Note that the enzyme is correctly named as a *dehydrogenase* named for the <u>more reduced</u> molecule. Now the first goal of the shuttle, the regeneration of cytosolic NAD$^+$ for glycolysis, has been completed.

Figure 2.19: The glycerol phosphate shuttle.

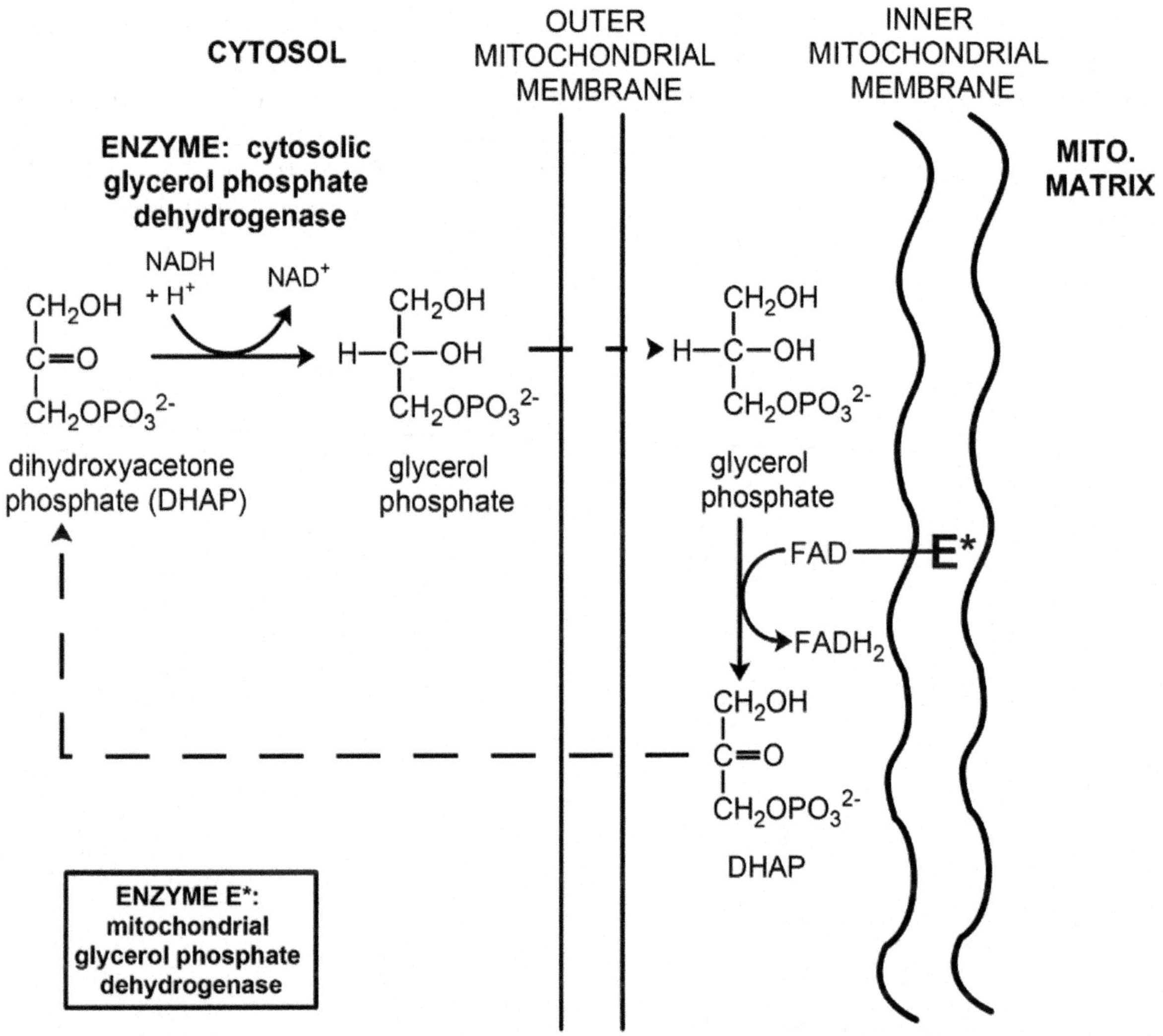

[<u>NOTE</u>: Start with **<u>dihydroxyacetone phosphate</u>** in the cytosol.]

Glycerol phosphate now moves into the intermembrane space of the mitochondria. Note that glycerol phosphate does not cross the mitochondrial inner membrane to go into the matrix. The mitochondrial glycerol phosphate dehydrogenase is embedded in the outer face of the mitochondrial inner membrane. It oxidizes glycerol phosphate back to dihydroxyacetone phosphate, which goes back to the cytosol. However, the mitochondrial glycerol phosphate dehydrogenase uses **FAD** as its coenzyme and reduces it to **FADH$_2$**. The use of FAD for this reaction is an exception to the "general rule" for when to use FAD, but serves a key purpose for this shuttle. The electrons of this FADH$_2$ are passed directly to coenzyme Q, an important intermediate of the electron transport chain, and thus are used for ATP synthesis—the second goal of the shuttle.

For the glycerol phosphate shuttle, the "net" conversion of cytosolic NADH to mitochondrial FADH$_2$ seems to waste about 1 ATP. The advantage of this shuttle, though, is that it allows the electrons from cytosolic NADH to be transported to the mitochondria against an NADH concentration gradient. The transport of the electrons from cytosolic NADH against the concentration gradient is especially important in actively metabolizing muscle tissue. In actively metabolizing tissues, the catabolic processes occurring in the mitochondria are producing much more NADH than is being produced by glycolysis in the cytosol.

CHAPTER 3: MITOCHONDRION OVERVIEW, THE PYRUVATE DEHYDROGENASE COMPLEX, AND THE TCA CYCLE

Objectives:

1. Explain the purpose of the pyruvate dehydrogenase complex, and why it is a key regulatory point of metabolism.

   a. Identify the aerobic and anaerobic fates of pyruvate.

2. Identify where the pyruvate dehydrogenase complex is located in the cell.

3. Explain the overall reaction steps (as fits the oxidation state pattern of metabolism) of the pyruvate dehydrogenase complex, and how certain vitamin deficiencies would affect this complex.

   a. Identify the two main steps of the pyruvate dehydrogenase complex as applications of the oxidation states basic principles.

   b. Identify the 3 catalytic components of the pyruvate dehydrogenase complex and each of their cofactors, and their vitamin precursors.

4. Explain when the PDH complex is activated or inhibited.

   a. Explain the regulation of the pyruvate dehydrogenase complex in terms of both of its regulatory components (the inhibitors and activators of the complex) and how it is hormonally controlled.

5. Define the process of the TCA cycle.

6. Explain the purpose of the TCA cycle.

   a. Describe the role of the TCA cycle in energy production.

7. Identify where the TCA cycle takes place in the cell.

8. Explain how the TCA cycle is carried out in the cell, and how vitamin deficiencies would affect this pathway.

   a. Name and recognize the structures of the starting products, key intermediates, and the end products of the TCA cycle.

   b. Name the 8 enzymes involved in the TCA cycle and describe the reactions they catalyze.

   c. Identify the four reactions of the TCA cycle where reducing equivalents are produced.

    d. Identify the products "per turn" of the TCA cycle, and be able to differentiate why glucose fuels 2 turns but alanine can only fuel 1 turn of the TCA cycle.

9. Explain when the TCA cycle occurs.

    a. Identify the regulatory enzymes of the TCA cycle; and how intermediates can be used for other synthetic processes; and how anaplerotic reactions can replenish TCA cycle intermediates.

10. Explain how a thiamine deficiency will affect the PDH complex and the TCA cycle, and why it would cause elevated levels of pyruvate and lactate in the blood.

MITOCHONDRIA: Structure and function

To get the maximum energy yield of ATP from glucose (30 to 32 ATP), pyruvate must be transported into the mitochondria, a cellular organelle. There the pyruvate will be completely oxidized to CO_2, and will make more reducing power (NADH and $FADH_2$) in the process. The reducing power will be used by the electron transport chain to produce a proton gradient. The proton gradient (i.e. electrical energy) will then be converted to chemical energy in the form of ATP.

A mitochondrion is about one micron in size, which is about the size of an *E. coli* bacterium (see **Figure 3.1**). A mitochondrion has an inner and outer membrane, the inner membrane space, and the matrix. The outer membrane of a mitochondrion contains pores, which are voltage dependent anion channels. These pores are permeable to many small molecules including ATP, ADP and many metabolites. The inner membrane space, between the two membranes of the mitochondrion, is where the protons are going to be pumped by the electron transport chain.

Figure 3.1: Basic structure of a mitochondrion

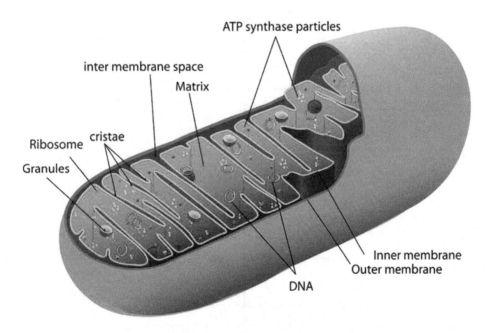

Mariana Ruiz Villarreal / Copyright in the Public Domain

The inner membrane is highly folded and forms a series of internal ridges referred to as cristae. These cristae can extend across the mitochondrial matrix to essentially create separate compartments within the matrix. All five complexes of the electron transport chain are also located in the inner membrane.

The inner membrane is impermeable to nearly all ions and polar molecules. If the inner membrane will not let protons freely flow across the membrane, nothing else is going to go across either. Thus anything that is allowed to cross the inner membrane is controlled, and will have to have some sort of transporter located in the inner membrane (as shown in **Figure 3.2**). **Figure 3.2** shows examples of the concept that anything that crosses the inner mitochondrial membrane, outlined here, needs a specific transporter. Think of the transporters as a "door." If the membrane is going to open the door to let a molecule out, then it also lets a molecule in. The organelle maximizes the use of the energy required to open that door.

Figure 3.2: Inner membrane transporters.

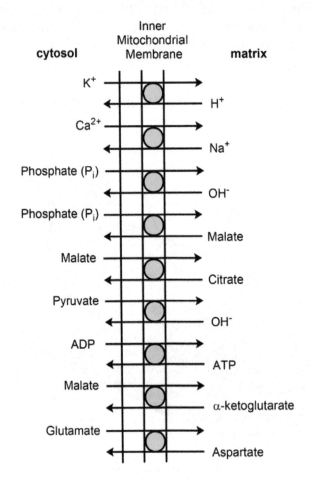

Various inner membrane transporters control the flow of essential molecules into and out of the matrix. The primary goal of these inner membrane transporters is to establish or maintain the membrane potential.

Thus, there is always a pair of molecules that can pass through the door. When one of those transporters (i.e. doors) opens, a molecule will exit the mitochondrium and a molecule will come into the mitochondrial matrix. Malate is a molecule that is allowed to cross the inner membrane, and has a several transporters that let it in or out of the matrix. Aspartate, glutamate and α-ketoglutarate are allowed to cross, and are key transporters of the malate-aspartate shuttle involved in regenerating cytosolic NAD+ for glycolysis. Notice, though, that oxaloacetate, NADH and NAD+ are not listed anywhere in the diagram. These molecules are not allowed to cross the inner membrane. There are numerous ion transporters, as well. The primary goal of these transporters is to establish or maintain the membrane potential, as well as transport intermediates necessary for various metabolic pathways.

The matrix of the mitochondrion, the center region of the organelle, carries out many pathways. Mitochondria are primarily catabolic organelles, as the primary function of mitochondria is the production of ATP using the reducing power generated by the breakdown (catabolism) of many molecules. The pyruvate dehydrogenase (PDH) complex and the tricarboxylic acid (TCA) cycle are located in mitochondria. The TCA cycle is the common destination of intermediates from the catabolism of carbohydrates, proteins, and lipids. Fatty acid oxidation is another breakdown (catabolic) pathway in the matrix. There are, however, some synthetic pathways in the matrix. These include ketone body synthesis, heme synthesis, and steroid synthesis. Some pathways actually "bridge" the mitochondrion. Part of the pathway will be in the mitochondria and part will take place in the cytosol. For example, gluconeogenesis is a synthetic pathway. The initial reactions of gluconeogenesis are actually in the mitochondria, while the remainder of the pathway is in the cytosol. As a result of the numerous pathways, the matrix has a very high concentration of proteins. The mitochondrion also has its own genome (located in the matrix). There are various diseases that occur in humans due to mutations in the mitochondrial genome.

Mitochondria use greater than 90% of the oxygen we breathe, as oxygen is the terminal electron acceptor of the electron transport chain. Oxygen is needed by all of the mitochondria because the mitochondria produce greater than 90% of all the ATP, which is the major function of the mitochondria. All of the catabolic pathways in the mitochondria, i.e. the TCA cycle, fatty acid oxidation, etc., send all of their NADH and FADH$_2$ to the electron transport chain to regenerate the oxidized form of those molecules (NAD+ and FAD). If the electron transport chain is not working, the cell does not run the TCA cycle or fatty acid oxidation because there is nowhere for all that reducing power to go. Glycolysis is the single *catabolic* pathway that will produce ATP, without relying on the electron transport chain to regenerate its cytosolic NAD+. Thus, it is very important that glycolysis is **not** in the mitochondria. When cells are lacking oxygen, glycolysis produces ATP for the cell by anaerobic glycolysis. Mature red blood cells, for instance, lack mitochondria and can only produce ATP via anaerobic glycolysis. Since the purpose of red blood cells is to transport oxygen to other cells and tissues, it is important that they do not use what they are transporting.

THE PYRUVATE DEHYDROGENASE COMPLEX: The bridging step between glycolysis and the TCA cycle

The pyruvate dehydrogenase (PDH) complex is the ***irreversible*** bridging step between glycolysis and the TCA cycle, which take place in the cytosol and the mitochondria respectively. Recall that α-keto acids are stable, such that the carboxylic acid group does not readily leave the molecule. Therefore, decarboxylating an α-keto acid is mechanistically "hard" or complex. Presented here is a _very_ simplified mechanism. It is not the actual mechanism. The intermediate drawn is "fake." The point is to draw the reactions so that they line up with what one has learned in the basic recipe of metabolism (**Figure 1.7** of chapter 1). The PDH complex is a multi-enzyme complex that converts pyruvate into acetyl CoA. Acetyl CoA is a structure one must know (recognize it and be able to draw the 2 carbon part—not the CoA part). The PDH complex is the irreversible bridge between glycolysis and the TCA cycle. Humans can convert sugars to fat, but cannot convert fatty acids back to sugar. In gluconeogenesis, the pyruvate is formed from non-carbohydrate precursors—not acetyl CoA. Pyruvate, for gluconeogenesis, comes from lactate, alanine or from the catabolism of other amino acids that will produce pyruvate. Thus, gluconeogenesis starts with pyruvate, not acetyl CoA.

The PDH complex can be defined (i.e. What?) as a multienzyme complex that converts pyruvate (a 3 carbon molecule) to acetyl-CoA (a 2 carbon unit attached to Coenzyme A) for entry into the TCA cycle under _aerobic_ conditions. The net reaction for the PDH complex is shown in **Figure 3.3**. The products of the PDH complex are acetyl CoA, NADH, and CO_2. The reason the reaction is irreversible, is due to the negative ΔG°' equal to – 8 kcal/mol for the net reaction of the complex. For a ΔG of a reaction that is equal to – 4 kcal/mol, or is more negative than – 4 kcal/mol, there is essentially nothing the cell can do to manipulate the ratio of products to reactants to make the reaction go in the other direction. Thus it is an irreversible reaction. In biological systems, though, certain irreversible reactions must be bypassed in some manner (i.e. gluconeogenesis bypassing the three irreversible reactions of glycolysis, as an example). The PDH complex, however, is an irreversible reaction that is not bypassed by another set of reactions.

Figure 3.3: Net reaction of the PDH complex

1 pyruvate + CoA + NAD^+ ⟶ 1 acetyl CoA + CO_2 + NADH   ΔG°' = -8 kcal/mol

The purpose of the PDH complex (i.e. Why?) is to decarboxylate pyruvate to form CO_2. The formation of CO_2 allows for the excretion of the first carbons from the breakdown of glucose (or other monosaccharides like fructose and galactose) or from the breakdown of certain amino acids. The PDH complex also produces NADH, as shown in the net reaction in **Figure 3.3**. This NADH is formed in the mitochondrial matrix, which is where the complex is located, so it can go directly to the ETC for energy production. The ETC will then regenerate mitochondrial NAD^+ for the pathways located in the matrix.

How does the PDH complex work? Again, think of this whole series of reactions as "hard" because it is decarboxylating an α-keto acid. The actual enzyme complex is large and contains five different enzymes, three catalytic and two regulatory. **Table 3.1** indicates the names of the three catalytic components of the complex, though they are often simply referred to as E_1, E_2, and E_3. In naming enzymes, anytime an enzyme (or enzyme complex) carries out multiple reactions, if one of the reactions is a redox reaction using NAD^+ or FAD, then the enzyme is called a dehydrogenase. Dehydrogenases are named for the more reduced molecule. However, the actual reduced molecule of the oxidation-reduction reaction of the complex is an intermediate attached lipoamide. Therefore, the enzyme name just uses the starting material of the complex, pyruvate. Hence the name of this enzyme complex is the pyruvate dehydrogenase complex. In fact, the first catalytic enzyme component is called pyruvate dehydrogenase.

Table 3.1: The three PDH complex catalytic enzymes and their overall reactions

Enzyme	Abbreviation	Prosthetic Group	Reaction Catalyzed
Pyruvate dehydrogenase component	E_1	TPP (Thiamine Pyrophosphate)	Oxidative decarboxylation of pyruvate
Dihydrolipoyl transacetylase	E_2	Lipoamide	Transfer of the acetyl group to CoA
Dihydrolipoyl dehydrogenase	E_3	FAD	Regeneration of the oxidized form of lipoamide

Each of the three catalytic enzymes has a prosthetic group associated with it (see **Table 3.1**). A prosthetic group is a coenzyme that is permanently associated with an enzyme. While a simplified reaction scheme for the complex will be drawn, knowing the prosthetic groups of each of the catalytic subunits is important. These prosthetic groups (coenzymes) are derived from vitamins. Thus certain vitamin deficiencies will affect the function of this complex, especially as it requires a number of coenzymes to function, as indicated in the chart. The first one is thiamine pyrophosphate, which is derived from the vitamin thiamine (vitamin B_1). Lipoamide is not a vitamin because the body actually makes it. However, FAD is derived from the vitamin riboflavin (B_2). Coenzyme A is part of the product of the complex, acetyl CoA. Coenzyme A is derived from the vitamin pantothenic acid (B_5). The vitamin niacin (B_3) is needed to produce the coenzyme nicotinamide adenine dinucleotide (NAD^+), which will be reduced to produce NADH + H^+. A deficiency in thiamine, riboflavin, or niacin will affect the ability of the PDH complex to function, as well as the α-ketoglutarate dehydrogenase complex of the TCA cycle because its mechanism is the same as the PDH complex.

Table 3.1 indicates the overall reaction catalyzed by the component. Note that E_3 has nothing to do with converting pyruvate to acetyl CoA. Lipoamide of E_2 is reduced as the product of the E_1 reaction, and the purpose of E_3 is to re-oxidize the lipoamide. Thus the complex catalyzes a series of oxidation-reduction reactions, as well as the decarboxylation that takes place at E_1. For the catalytic reaction of E_3, its prosthetic group FAD gets reduced to $FADH_2$. This $FADH_2$ cannot go to the electron transport chain because it is permanently attached to E_2. For the whole complex to function again, the $FADH_2$ of E_3 needs to be re-oxidized back to FAD. Thus this is where NAD^+ is reduced to $NADH + H^+$. This NADH is not attached to the complex and does carry electrons to the electron transport chain.

The advantage of having all of these enzymes together in a single complex enhances the rate of the sequential reactions and minimizes the side reactions that could occur. The organization of the enzymes into a complex also serves to stabilize against proteolysis, the breakdown of the enzyme itself. Coordinated regulation is also permitted by this organization of enzymes, as all of the reactions need to occur or none of them. Again, this is an irreversible step between glycolysis and the TCA cycle, so regulation of the complex is very important.

Figure 3.4: The PDH complex reaction as two main steps (as applies to the "Oxidation States" Flow Chart).

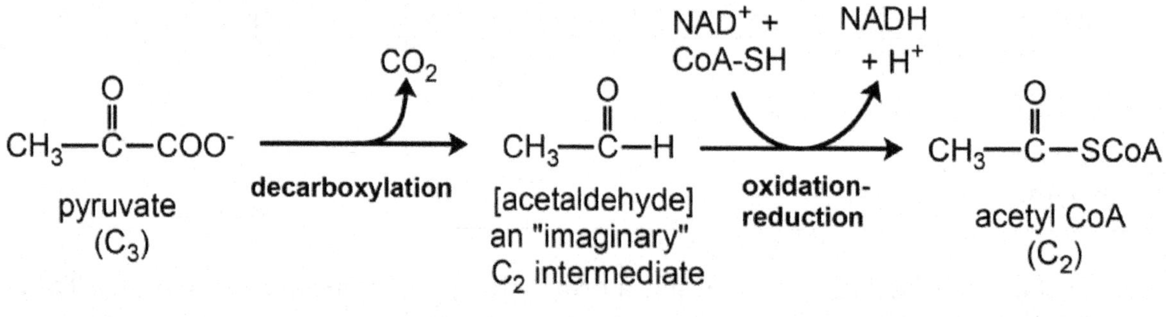

Note: The real mechanism is much more complex. The main point is that α-keto acids are able to be decarboxylated, but require a complex mechanistic reaction sequence.

Figure 3.4 is the simplified reaction sequence carried out by the PDH complex. It is divided into a two-step reaction. We have a carboxylic acid group on pyruvate, with a keto group in the alpha position. The first step is to decarboxylate pyruvate, to yield what I will call an "imaginary" or "fake" intermediate, acetaldehyde. The aldehyde group would be formed if the intermediate were to be released. In actuality the intermediate is attached to the lipoamide coenzyme of E_2, so the aldehyde functionality is not really formed.

In this simplified reaction scheme: the first step is decarboxylation and the second step is a redox reaction. This two-step reaction scheme will account for all of the products of the PDH complex. Following the oxidation states flow chart, after the decarboxylation forms the aldehyde the complex oxidizes it. Oxidation of an aldehyde yields a carboxylic acid, but in this case the carboxylic acid gets attached to coenzyme A to form a thioester. A thioester function is equivalent in its oxidation state to a carboxylic acid. So attaching the acetaldehyde at the aldehyde carbon to CoA elevates it in oxidation state to the oxidation state of a carboxylic acid. Another way to look at it is if the CoA were to be clipped off by adding water across the thioester bond, the product would be acetate (a two carbon fatty acid).

As noted in the discussion of the three catalytic enzymes, the real mechanism is much more complex. However, this simple two-step reaction sequence follows the "rules" of the oxidation flow chart and accounts for all the products of the complex. Oxidation and reduction reactions are always coupled. According the "rules", NAD^+ is used when oxidizing from an aldehyde to an acid, which accounts for the product NADH + H^+. [The real reaction series involves the oxidation and reduction of two other prosthetic groups, lipoamide and FAD.] It is the NADH that is formed, though, that is able to carry electrons to the electron transport chain. The PDH complex decarboxylates pyruvate forming CO_2, acetyl CoA, and NADH. These are the products of this complex, and the starting and ending materials of pyruvate and acetyl CoA are two key structures one should know.

This simplified two-step reaction scheme will be shown again with the α-ketoglutarate complex in the TCA cycle. The mechanism is the same because the complex is also decarboxylating an α-keto acid, exactly like the PDH complex. However, the α-ketoglutarate complex does not have the same regulatory subunits on it. It does have the same prosthetic groups, the same enzyme mechanism, and the product is also attached to CoA.

Regulation of pathways is very complex. Control of metabolic pathways is often more dependent on the overall ratio of key regulators rather than the absolute amounts of any given regulator. In this text, regulation of pathways and enzymes will be covered to emphasize several major concepts of regulation. The first is that coordinated regulation of pathways often includes the reversible phosphorylation of key enzymes. The PDH complex has two regulatory enzymes the control the phosphorylation state of E_1 (the pyruvate dehydrogenase component), as expected as that is where the reaction series starts. The two regulatory enzymes of the PDH complex are the pyruvate dehydrogenase kinase and the pyruvate dehydrogenase phosphatase. Recall that kinases are enzymes that phosphorylate something and are named after what they phosphorylate. Thus the pyruvate dehydrogenase kinase phosphorylates pyruvate dehydrogenase (E_1). Phosphorylation of E_1 turns *off* the complex. Removal of this phosphate group by the pyruvate dehydrogenase phosphatase would then turn on the PDH complex. Note the phosphatase is named after what it dephosphorylates.

Insulin and glucagon are two hormones that control the phosphorylation state of the PDH complex in their respective target tissues (as well as key enzymes in other metabolic pathways) to achieve coordinated control of these metabolic pathways. Insulin is the hormone that indicates blood glucose is plenty, and thus cells can take up glucose as needed to carry out metabolic pathways. Insulin is considered an activator of synthetic pathways, since glucose is readily available as an energy source through its catabolism or for use in synthetic pathways and to replenish glycogen stores for certain cells/tissues. Glucagon, on the other hand, indicates low blood sugar and is responsible for targeting the liver (primarily) resulting in the release of glucose into the blood from the liver either from liver glycogen stores or from gluconeogenesis (*de novo* synthesis of glucose).

One should consider what enzymes should be on or off in the liver when insulin is the predominant hormone in the blood versus glucagon. The liver is the organ responsible for sensing the nutrient needs of the body and supplying them. The liver is a major target tissue for both insulin and glucagon. For instance for the PDH complex, which hormone would active it, and which hormone would inactivate the complex? If insulin is the predominant hormone, glucose is readily available. The liver would respond by replenishing its glycogen stores; doing glycolysis, the TCA cycle, and the ETC to raise its ATP levels in the cells; and to store excess glucose as fats, which requires glycolysis, the PDH complex and the first step of the TCA cycle prior to doing fatty acid synthesis. Insulin would activate the PDH complex under these conditions. Insulin would, therefore, activate the pyruvate dehydrogenase phosphatase to remove the phosphate from E_1 to turn on the complex.

When glucagon is the predominant hormone, the liver will begin by releasing glucose into the blood from its glycogen stores. If the stores are not sufficient, then glucose will be made *de novo* from pyruvate via gluconeogenesis. If gluconeogenesis is activated to help replenish blood glucose levels, then the PDH complex needs to be off (as the pyruvate carboxylase enzyme of gluconeogenesis is on). Thus glucagon activates the PDH complex kinase to phosphorylate E_1 of the PDH complex to turn it off.

Another key regulatory concept one should consider is the ratio of the cellular concentration of ATP versus ADP or AMP. If the concentration of ATP is high in the cell, the cell is generally doing synthetic processes, not catabolic processes. The PDH complex would generally be inhibited by high ATP concentrations, and activated by high AMP concentrations.

A third key regulatory concept involves two enzymes in the same cellular compartment that use the same substrate. In mitochondria there are two enzymes that utilize pyruvate as a substrate, the pyruvate dehydrogenase complex and pyruvate carboxylase. These two enzymes are not on simultaneously (in general) in the mitochondria. Again the focus is on the liver, as a primary example. If the liver is doing gluconeogenesis, which involves pyruvate carboxylase, the PDH complex needs to be off. To achieve this control, acetyl CoA inhibits the PDH complex and activates pyruvate carboxylase. Thus control of two enzymes is achieved with one molecule. One can simply attribute acetyl CoA as "product inhibition" of the PDH complex. High concentrations of acetyl CoA could result if the TCA cycle is slowing down because the cell has plenty of ATP. If the ETC is off, the concentrations of NADH build up in the cell leading to the inhibition of the TCA cycle and ultimately the PDH complex because the acetyl CoA is not entering the TCA cycle. However, in particular in the liver, a high concentration of acetyl CoA generally comes from beta-oxidation of fatty acids (not the PDH complex, itself), and the acetyl CoA will be used for ketone body synthesis (rather than go into the TCA cycle) under those conditions. The importance of acetyl CoA as a regulator of pyruvate carboxylase and the PDH complex will be discussed in more detail when covering the lipid pathways.

Again, the PDH complex is a bridging step and a key regulatory point for the fate of pyruvate. The conversion of pyruvate to acetyl CoA is irreversible, and in humans the fatty acids cannot be converted back to sugars. Thus, the conversion of glucose ultimately to acetyl CoA (i.e. the PDH complex is on) typically commits acetyl CoA molecules to one of two paths. They may enter the TCA cycle to burn off the two carbons of the acetyl CoA as CO_2 and produce more reducing power in the form of NADH and $FADH_2$ for the ETC for energy production. Or the acetyl CoA may be used for lipid synthesis (i.e. fatty acids for triacylglycerides or membrane lipids, or cholesterol). If the PDH complex is off, pyruvate formed from glycolysis will be used for lactate production (i.e. anaerobic glycolysis) or for amino acid synthesis, like alanine. If pyruvate is converted to oxaloacetate by pyruvate carboxylase in the mitochondria, then gluconeogenesis is occurring and the cell is making glucose, and the PDH complex is off under these conditions.

THE TRICARBOXYLIC ACID (TCA) CYCLE

The tricarboxylic acid (TCA) cycle is a pathway that will truly demonstrate all of the principles covered in the oxidation states chapter of this book. This pathway will provide a concrete example of how to understand a pathway by applying the oxidation states flow chart (i.e. basic recipe of metabolism), as well as the enzyme naming rules.

Figure 3.5: The **net** reaction of the TCA cycle.

$$1 \text{ acetyl CoA} + 3 \text{ NAD}^+ + \text{FAD} + \text{GDP} + P_i + 2 \text{ H}_2\text{O} \longrightarrow 2 \text{ CO}_2 + 3 \text{ NADH} + \text{FADH}_2 + \text{GTP} + 2 \text{ H}^+ + \text{CoA}$$

These are the products "per turn" of the TCA cycle.

As this pathway is a cycle, one should learn the products of the pathway "per cycle" or "per turn" of the cycle as shown in the net reaction of **Figure 3.5**. The catabolic pathways of various biological molecules funnel intermediates into the TCA cycle. Thus one should know which reactions produce the products of the cycle, and that the entry of acetyl CoA into the cycle yields all of the products, will help in understanding the energy yields obtained from the catabolism of various nutrients. For example, a molecule of glucose will ultimately "turn" the TCA cycle two times (i.e. from two molecules of acetyl CoA), but a fatty acid will turn the TCA cycle many times (i.e. palmitate, a C_{16} fatty acid, will turn it 8 times).

For the net reaction of the TCA cycle (**Figure 3.5**), the entry of acetyl CoA into the pathway is considered the start of the cycle. The pathway begins, then, with the entry of acetyl CoA, a two carbon unit. The products of the TCA cycle include two CO_2 molecules. Those exact two carbons of the acetyl CoA entering the cycle are not burned off in a single turn of the cycle. It usually takes a couple turns to burn off those two specific carbons. The focus here, though, is not on the actual mechanisms—rather the pattern. Thus, two carbons are coming into the cycle, and two carbons are burned off. Acetyl CoA, then, cannot yield a glucose molecule. The PDH complex is irreversible, and the entry of acetyl CoA into the TCA burns off two carbons prior to the formation of oxaloacetate. Also the formation of oxaloacetate for gluconeogenesis comes from pyruvate via pyruvate carboxylase, not acetyl CoA. Thus the cell cannot achieve net synthesis of glucose from a molecule of acetyl CoA. The TCA cycle also yields four molecules of reducing power (3 NADH and 1 $FADH_2$), which go to the electron transport chain, along with 1 GTP (energy equivalent) directly, some protons and a molecule of coenzyme A.

To define the TCA cycle (What?): The TCA cycle completes the oxidation of the acetyl unit (the two carbon portion) of acetyl CoA to CO_2, and serves as the final common pathway for the oxidation of fuel molecules (amino acids, fatty acids, and carbohydrates). After the two molecules of pyruvate from glycolysis have been converted to two molecules of acetyl CoA, there are now four carbons left from the original glucose molecule. These four carbons need to be oxidized to the level of a carboxylic acid so they can be clipped off as CO_2 to completely burn off the six carbons of glucose. These two molecules of acetyl CoA formed from glucose will "turn" the TCA cycle two times. By the end of two turns of the TCA cycle, four CO_2 molecules will be formed, essentially completing the complete oxidation of glucose. [Note, though, that one turn of the TCA cycle does not clip off the same two carbons from the entering acetyl unit.] The catabolism of fatty acids and amino acids also feed into various points in the TCA cycle to completely oxidize the carbon backbones, or to provide intermediates for other synthetic pathways. This pathway occurs when *oxygen is present* because all of the reducing power needs to go to the electron transport chain for ATP generation.

The TCA cycle has several important purposes (Why?). The TCA cycle is responsible for one of the main mechanisms of excreting carbons as CO_2, with two molecules of CO_2 formed per turn of the cycle. One turn of the TCA cycle also yields one GTP, which is equivalent in energy to an ATP, and four molecules of reducing power (3 NADH and 1 $FADH_2$), which are the electron donors for the ETC for the formation of ATP. Some of the TCA intermediates can also be used for anabolic (synthetic) processes. Thus the TCA cycle is considered an amphibolic pathway, meaning it serves both catabolic and anabolic functions, and it takes place in the mitochondrial matrix (Where?). To be absolutely specific, the succinate dehydrogenase enzyme of the TCA cycle is actually part of Complex II of the ETC in the inner mitochondrial membrane.

How the TCA cycle proceeds is shown completely in **Figure 3.6**, but each step will be covered individually. The cycle is divided into eight steps based on the eight enzymes of the cycle. Some of the enzymes carry out more than one reaction, though. After the steps have been covered individually, one should come back to look at the complete cycle to "walk" through the entire cycle or draw it out separately to ensure understanding of the reaction sequence, enzyme names, and coenzymes needed. **Figure 3.6** does indicate both actual intermediates, as well as some "fake" intermediates. All of the intermediates drawn are to emphasize how the pathway follows the oxidation states flow chart ("basic recipe of metabolism"). Always know starting and ending products, which for this pathway are acetyl CoA, oxaloacetate, and citrate. Remember none of these steps are explaining the actual enzyme mechanisms, just emphasizing the pattern of the series of reactions.

Figure 3.6: The TCA cycle

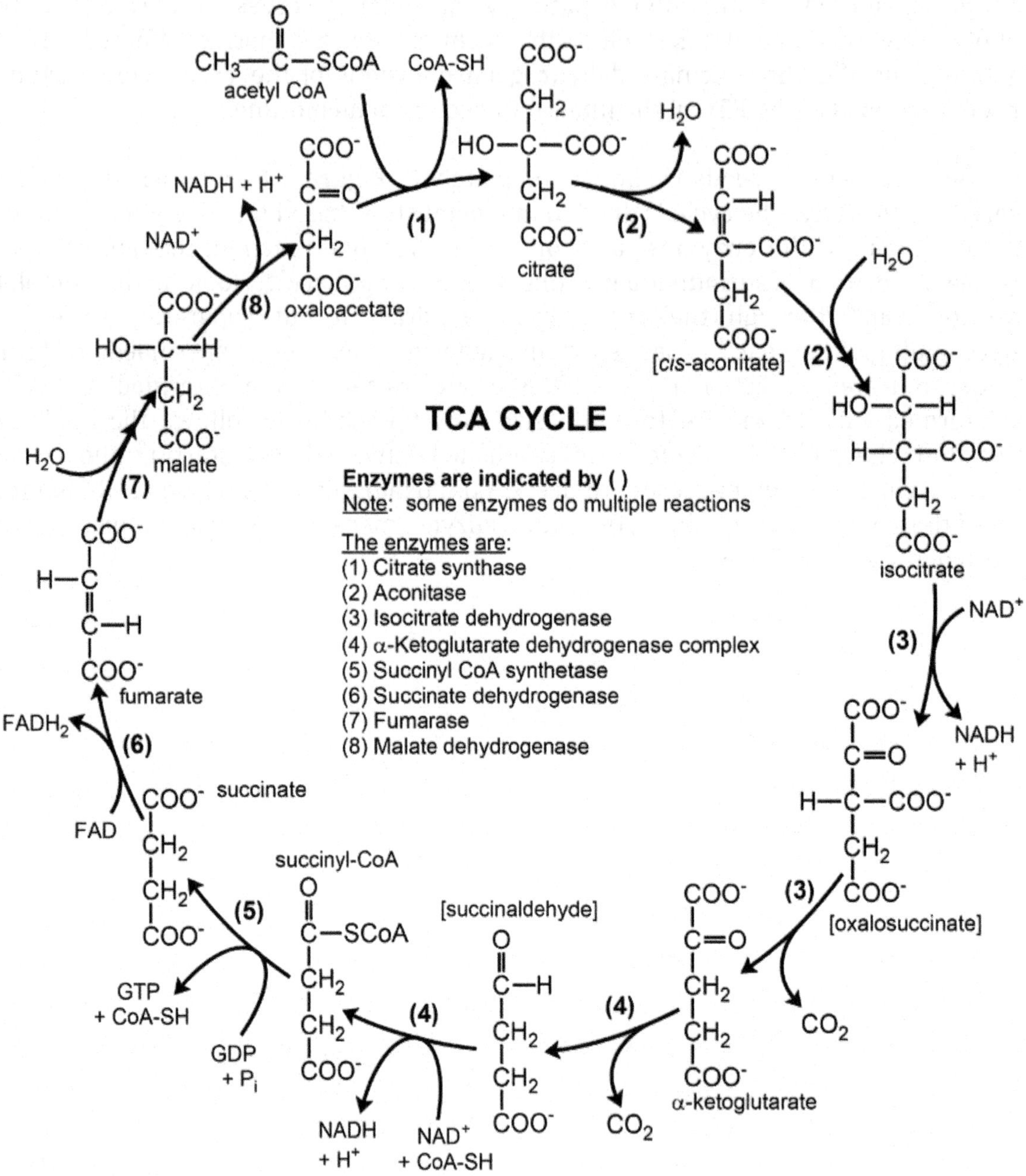

In the TCA cycle several of the enzymes carry out multiple reactions. Key intermediates in these enzymatic reactions are indicated by [ ]. These intermediates are specifically drawn, so correlations to the "Oxidation States Flow Chart" (**Figure 1.7**) and "Stability of carboxylic acids" (**Figure 1.14**) figures can be more readily seen.

Figure 3.7: STEP 1—Entry of acetyl CoA into the cycle by condensation with oxaloacetate

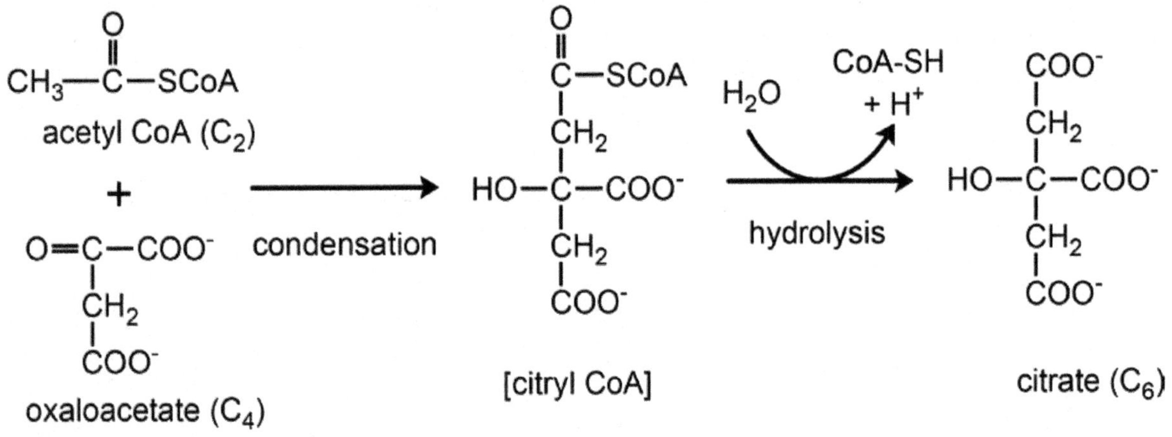

Enzyme: citrate synthase

Figure 3.7 shows the condensation reaction between the 4-carbon oxaloacetate and the 2 carbon unit of acetyl CoA to make the 6 carbon citrate. Citrate is also known as tricarboxylic acid (TCA), due to the three carboxylic acid groups on it, giving the pathway its name. The molecule of oxaloacetate is drawn "bent" in **Figure 3.7** to emphasize which carbons are attached between the two molecules. The carbonyl carbon of oxaloacetate forms a covalent bond to the methyl carbon of acetyl CoA, such that the entire acetyl CoA molecule is attached to oxaloacetate forming the intermediate citryl CoA. Water is used to cleave off coenzyme A, which now has a free thiol (-SH) group. This hydrolysis of citryl CoA pulls the overall reaction far in the direction of forming citrate. Note that citrate can also be used as the transporter of the "acetyl unit" to the cytosol for fatty acid synthesis, as will be discussed when covering that pathway.

This is a synthesis reaction in a catabolic pathway. Enzymes that synthesize molecules are either named as a *synthase* (no energy required) or *synthetase* (energy required). Then place the name of the **product** before synthase or synthetase. Since no energy is required in this reaction, the enzyme is called ***citrate synthase***.

In the 5-carbon "straight chain" part of citrate, notice the middle carbon is attached to **three** carbons and a hydroxyl group. Thus, this part of the molecule is a tertiary alcohol and CANNOT be further oxidized because one of the carbon-carbon bonds would have to be broken such that two bonds can be made to the oxygen. This cannot be done unless they have good leaving groups attached. While one of the groups attached to this center carbon is a carboxylic acid, there must be a keto group nearby to get it to leave, which is not there—yet.

Citrate does have three carboxylic acid groups on it, and one goal of the TCA cycle is to remove two of them. In biological molecules, the removal of carboxylic acid groups as molecules of CO_2 requires a keto group alpha (α) or beta (β) to it. There is a hydroxy group on the molecule of citrate that could become a keto group if it was a secondary alcohol, rather than the tertiary alcohol it is currently. Therefore, to be able to oxidize this hydroxy group to a keto group, it needs to be moved off of that "center" carbon of citrate.

Figure 3.8: STEP 2—Isomerization of citrate to isocitrate

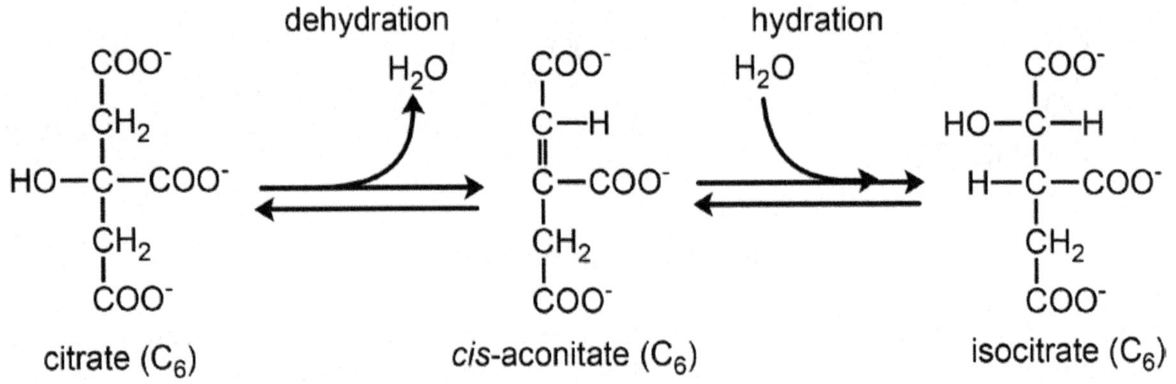

Enzyme: aconitase

Figure 3.8 shows the reaction sequence catalyzed by aconitase that "moves" the hydroxy group. Aconitase moves the hydroxy group first by a **dehydration** reaction to make the alkene intermediate *cis*-aconitate, followed by a **hydration** reaction where the –OH group is now on one of the "original" CH_2 carbons forming the product isocitrate. Recall from the oxidation states flow chart (**Figure 1.7**) that alkenes and alcohols are at the same oxidation state and can be interchanged by the addition or removal of an entire water molecule. This enzyme does that exact interchange, only now between a tertiary alcohol, an alkene, and a secondary alcohol. The hydroxy group is now a secondary alcohol on isocitrate, and can be oxidized to a ketone.

There are not specific rules for naming enzymes that carry out hydration and dehydration reactions. Although enzymes that specifically carry out hydration reactions are typically called hydratases. Enzymes that catalyze dehydration reactions are typically referred to as dehydratases. However, this enzyme carries out both a dehydration and hydration reaction. Thus, the enzyme *aconitase* is simply named after the intermediate in this reaction, *cis*-aconitate.

Figure 3.9: STEP 3—The first oxidation-reduction reaction of the cycle.

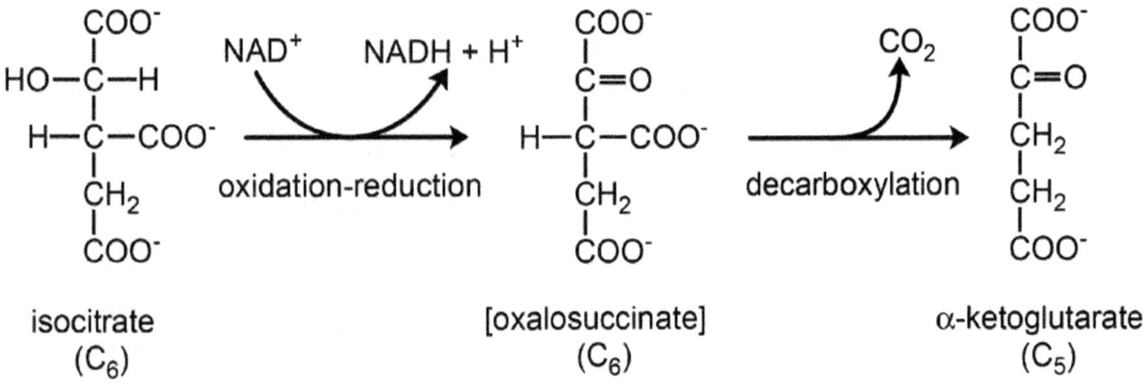

Enzyme: isocitrate dehydrogenase

Figure 3.9 shows the two reactions carried out by the enzyme isocitrate dehydrogenase, which catalyzes the first of four redox reactions of the TCA cycle. Isocitrate is first oxidized and then decarboxylated to form α-ketoglutarate. The first reaction is <u>oxidation</u> of the secondary alcohol group on isocitrate to a keto group to form the intermediate oxalosuccinate. If oxidation occurs, a molecule must be reduced because the hydrogens need to go onto another molecule. Since this oxidation is from an alcohol to a ketone, NAD⁺ is reduced to NADH + H⁺.

Notice the position of this keto group on oxalosuccinate relative to two out of the three carboxylic acid groups. The newly formed keto group is alpha (α) to one of the carboxyl groups (the top one in **Figure 3.9**) and beta (β) to a second carboxyl group (the one on the center carbon of the molecule). Beta-keto carboxylic acids are more unstable. Thus the carboxylic acid on the center carbon of oxalosuccinate will leave first.

The second reaction carried out by isocitrate dehydrogenase is <u>decarboxylation</u> (loss of CO_2) of that β-keto carboxyl group to get α-ketoglutarate, which is five carbons. While β-keto acids are unstable and spontaneously decarboxylate, spontaneous does not mean "instantaneous." Spontaneous does not indicate how long it will take for the carboxylic acid group to leave. Therefore, enzymes still typically carry out the decarboxylation of β-keto acids. Anytime an enzyme carries out more than one reaction, if one of the reactions is an oxidation-reduction reaction and (typically) uses NAD⁺ or FAD, the enzyme is called *dehydrogenase*. Dehydrogenases are named for the more <u>reduced</u> molecule, so this enzyme is called ***isocitrate dehydrogenase.***

The rate of α-ketoglutarate formation is important in determining the overall rate of the TCA cycle. The product, α-ketoglutarate, is also an amino acid precursor (or breakdown product) and can be converted to glutamate by a transamination reaction (**Figure 1.5**).

Figure 3.10: STEP 4—The second redox reaction of the cycle.

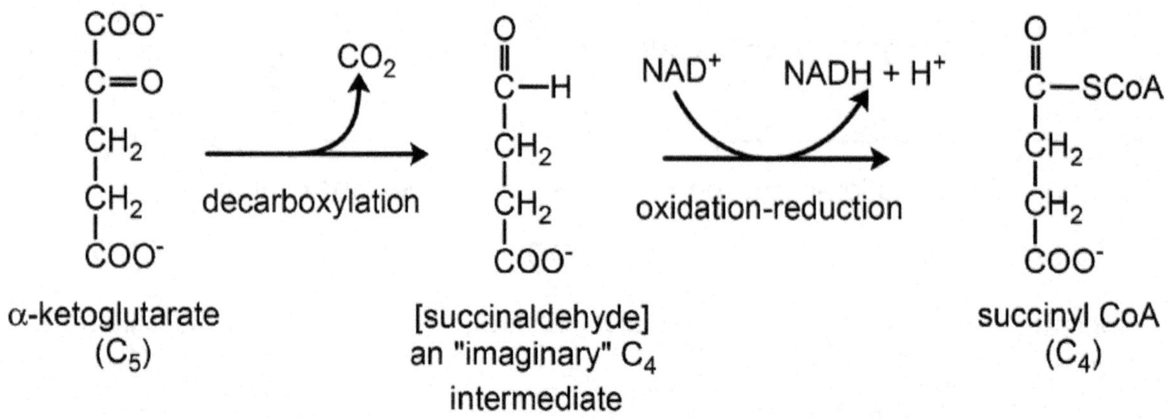

α-ketoglutarate (C$_5$) → decarboxylation → [succinaldehyde] an "imaginary" C$_4$ intermediate → oxidation-reduction → succinyl CoA (C$_4$)

Enzyme: α-ketoglutarate dehydrogenase complex
Shown as a simplified two-step reaction sequence of the α-ketoglutarate complex (as applies to the Oxidation States Flow Chart).

The α-ketoglutarate dehydrogenase complex reaction series shown in **Figure 3.10** is the "simplified" two-step reaction sequence that is exactly analogous to the PDH complex two-step mechanism shown in **Figure 3.4**. This is actually an enzyme complex, consisting of three catalytic enzymes, that carries out multiple reactions because the removal of an α-keto carboxylic acid is difficult, as seen for the decarboxylation of pyruvate. This complex is a regulated step of the TCA cycle. However, it does not have the kinase and phosphatase regulatory subunits like the PDH complex.

The complex does an oxidation-reduction reaction and a decarboxylation like isocitrate dehydrogenase, only in the reverse order. This time decarboxylation happens first to yield the intermediate succinaldehyde (a "fake" intermediate), which is 4 carbons. Then oxidation takes place, ultimately by the addition of coenzyme A, to form a thioester group, which is equivalent to the carboxylic acid group oxidation state. So the molecule has been oxidized from a 4 carbon aldehyde to the 4 carbon succinyl CoA. Again, NAD$^+$ is reduced to NADH + H$^+$ when oxidizing an aldehyde to a carboxylic acid.

For the naming of this enzyme complex, multiple reactions are being carried out. One of the reactions is an oxidation-reduction reaction using NAD$^+$ or FAD, so the enzyme complex is called a *dehydrogenase*. Dehydrogenases are named for the more reduced molecule. In this case the more reduced molecule is an intermediate that cannot be isolated, so the enzyme is named for the "initial" substrate for this enzyme: α-ketoglutarate. [Recall that the pyruvate dehydrogenase complex is named in a similar manner.]

The actual reaction mechanism for removing an α-keto carboxyl group is very similar to the pyruvate dehydrogenase complex, complete with final addition of CoA to the molecule (just like forming acetyl CoA). It requires three catalytic enzymes, which have the same prosthetic groups: thiamine pyrophosphate, lipoamide, and FAD. This reaction is very favorable and irreversible ($\Delta G^{o'}$ = - 8.0 kcal/mol). The products of the complex are CO_2, NADH, and succinyl CoA. Carbon dioxide is excreted, NADH is a substrate for the ETC, and succinyl CoA can be used for heme biosynthesis.

At this point in the TCA cycle, succinyl CoA is a four-carbon molecule. Of the original three carboxylic acid groups that were on the six-carbon citrate, two have been removed as CO_2. As the TCA cycle "ends" with the formation of the four-carbon oxaloacetate, no more carbons will be lost.

Figure 3.11: STEP 5—A substrate level phosphorylation which produces GTP.

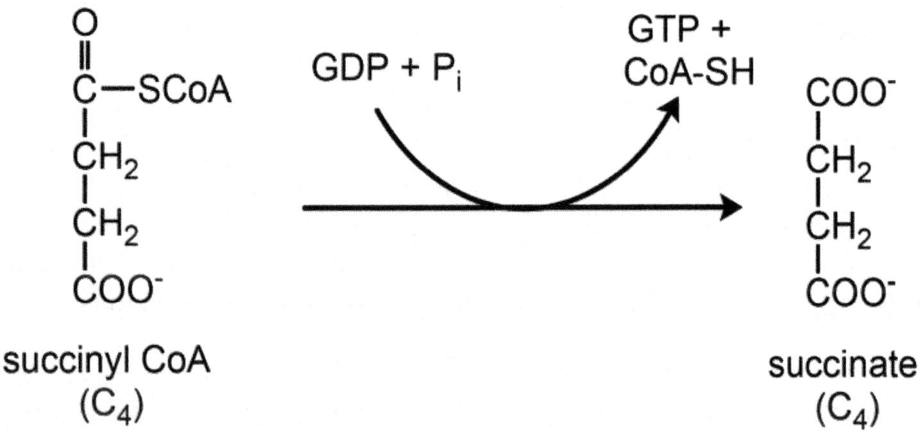

**Enzyme: succinyl CoA synthetase
(a.k.a. succinate thiokinase)**

Figure 3.11 shows the reaction carried out by succinyl CoA synthetase. This reaction is a substrate level phosphorylation, where the phosphorylation of GDP to make GTP occurs at the expense of a high-energy organic substrate, succinyl-CoA. The thioester bond of succinyl CoA is a high energy bond ($\Delta G^{o'}$ for the thioester hydrolysis is approximately -8.6 kcal/mol). Cleavage of this bond provides enough energy to drive the phosphorylation of GDP + P_i to make GTP (the phosphoanhydride bond created has approximately -7.3 kcal/mol). Note that succinyl-CoA has NO phosphate groups on it. Inorganic phosphate (P_i) is the donor of the phosphate. The product of this reaction is the four-carbon molecule succinate, and this reaction is readily reversible ($\Delta G^{o'}$ = -0.7 kcal/mol).

This enzyme is known as succinyl CoA synthetase or as succinate thiokinase. Both names of this enzyme are based on the *reverse* reaction, as if the energy from GTP is used to add coenzyme A to succinate to form succinyl CoA. For the name **succinyl CoA synthetase**, this enzyme is named as if succinyl CoA is being synthesized and the enzyme naming rules are more obviously applied. If you consider the reverse reaction, it would be a synthesis reaction that requires the use of energy. GTP is an energy equivalent to ATP. Thus name the enzyme a *synthetase* and use the name of the "product." Considering the reverse reaction, the product would be succinyl CoA. Therefore the enzyme is named succinyl CoA synthetase.

In naming the enzyme **succinate thiokinase**, the rules for naming kinases still apply. This enzyme is being named for the *reverse* reaction. In this case GTP is "donating" the **energy** this time (NOT the actual phosphate group) from cleaving the high-energy phosphate bond to creating the thioester bond of succinyl-CoA. Or more simply, a *thiokinase* is donating a thiol group to the acceptor molecule rather than the usual phosphate group of a typical kinase. Thus, succinate is still the "acceptor" of both the thiol group from coenzyme CoA and the energy from cleaving the phosphate bond to make it. Hence it is named succinate thiokinase.

This is the only step of the TCA cycle that directly produces a molecule of chemical energy, GTP. The name succinyl CoA synthetase, in the author's opinion, is a better name to help one remember the energy is produced in this step. GTP is, like ATP, a form of chemical energy used by cells. GTP is often used for protein synthesis, signal transduction processes (i.e. G-protein coupled receptors), and the γ-phosphate group can be transferred to ADP to form ATP by a nucleoside diphosphate kinase.

*The last three reactions regenerate oxaloacetate (C4) so that the cycle can continue. At this point, look at the differences in structure between the four-carbon succinate molecule (**Figure 3.11**) and the four-carbon oxaloacetate molecule. Notice that both have carboxylic acid groups at both ends of the molecule. However, the two "middle" carbons of succinate are at the level of an alkane; while one of the "middle" carbons of oxaloacetate has a keto group. To put that keto group on the molecule, the same sequence will be used as is outlined in the Oxidation States Flow Chart (**Figure 1.7**): 1) oxidize the alkane to an alkene; 2) hydrate to form a secondary alcohol; 3) oxidize to a ketone.*

Figure 3.12: STEP 6—The third redox reaction of the cycle.

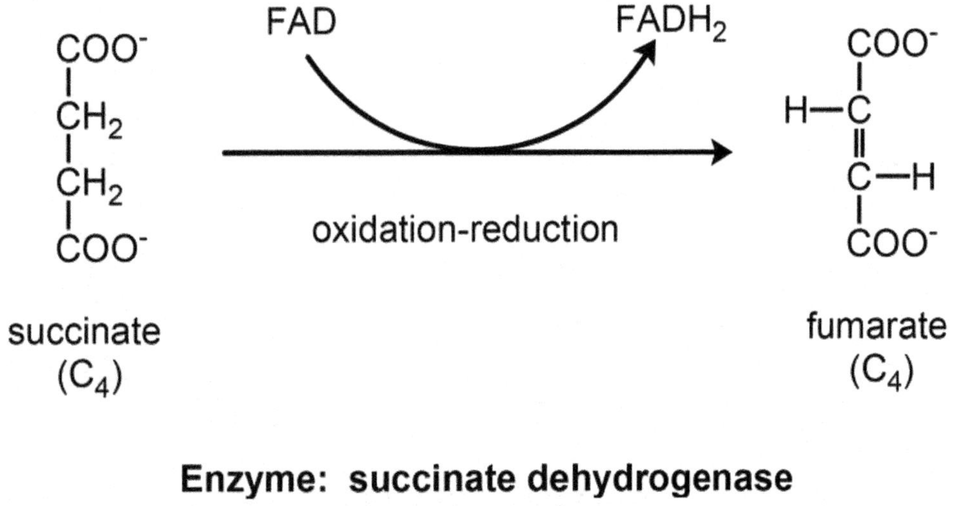

Enzyme: succinate dehydrogenase

Succinate dehydrogenase catalyzes the oxidation-reduction reaction shown in **Figure 3.12**. The two middle carbons of succinate are at the level of an alkane and are oxidized to the alkene of fumarate. Since the oxidation is occurring from the level of an alkane to an alkene, FAD is the acceptor of the hydrogens to be reduced to $FADH_2$. FAD is used here because the free energy change (ΔG) is not sufficient to reduce NAD^+. Enzymes that carry out oxidation-reduction reactions (and use NAD^+ or FAD) are called *dehydrogenases*. Dehydrogenases are named for the more <u>reduced</u> molecule, which for this reaction is succinate. Thus, the enzyme is called ***succinate dehydrogenase***.

The FAD used in this reaction is covalently attached to a histidine ring of the enzyme, meaning that it cannot dissociate from the enzyme. Succinate dehydrogenase, though, is actually part of Complex II of the ETC. Therefore the electrons of the $FADH_2$ formed in this reaction are transferred immediately to the electron transport chain.

Figure 3.13 shows the hydration reaction carried out by ***fumarate hydratase***, which is more commonly known as ***fumarase***. Fumarate is hydrated, the addition of an entire water molecule across the double bond, to form the secondary alcohol group on malate. Recall that alkenes and alcohols are at the same oxidation level, so this is not a redox reaction. If using the enzyme naming rules, hydratases are enzymes that add water to a molecule. Hydratases are typically named for the molecule to which the water molecule is added. In this case, fumarate hydratase is the more accurate enzyme name based on naming rules.

Figure 3.13: STEP 7—A hydration step to go from an alkene to a secondary alcohol.

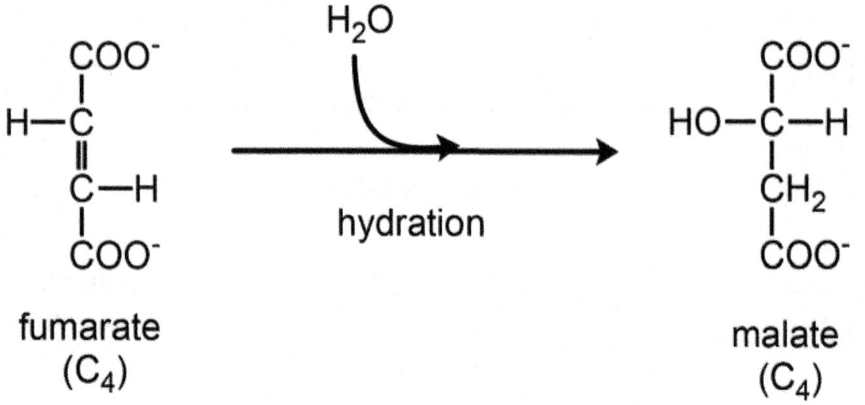

Enzyme: fumarase
(a.k.a. fumarate hydratase)

The "last" step of the cycle is the oxidation of malate (secondary alcohol group) to oxaloacetate (keto group), shown in **Figure 3.14**. Since the oxidation is occurring from a secondary alcohol to a ketone, NAD$^+$ is reduced to NADH + H$^+$. Again, enzymes that carry out redox reactions and use NAD$^+$ or FAD are called *dehydrogenases*. Dehydrogenases are named for the more <u>reduced</u> molecule, which is malate for this reaction. Thus, the enzyme is called ***malate dehydrogenase***.

The reaction for the formation of oxaloacetate is very endergonic and unfavorable. The $\Delta G^{o'}$ for this reaction, as written for the formation of oxaloacetate, is + 7 kcal/mol. Thus the reverse reaction, the formation of malate, has a $\Delta G^{o'}$ of -7 kcal/mol. The formation of malate by malate dehydrogenase should then be essentially an irreversible reaction, but it is not. Cells bypass irreversible reactions (if it is necessary) typically in one of two ways. The reverse reaction is a different reaction and uses different enzymes, as seen in gluconeogenesis for bypassing the three irreversible reactions of glycolysis. Or a reaction is coupled to a favorable reaction to make a reaction go in an unfavored direction, as free energies (ΔG) of reactions are additive. In this case, oxaloacetate is the product of one reaction and the substrate of the subsequent reaction. The key is to keep the malate concentration high and the oxaloacetate concentration in the mitochondria very low (i.e. as soon as it is formed, it is used) by its immediate use in the citrate synthase reaction, which is very favorable ($\Delta G^{o'}$ = -7.7 kcal/mol). Thus malate dehydrogenase continues to form oxaloacetate under these conditions.

Figure 3.14: STEP 8—The fourth redox reaction and completes the cycle.

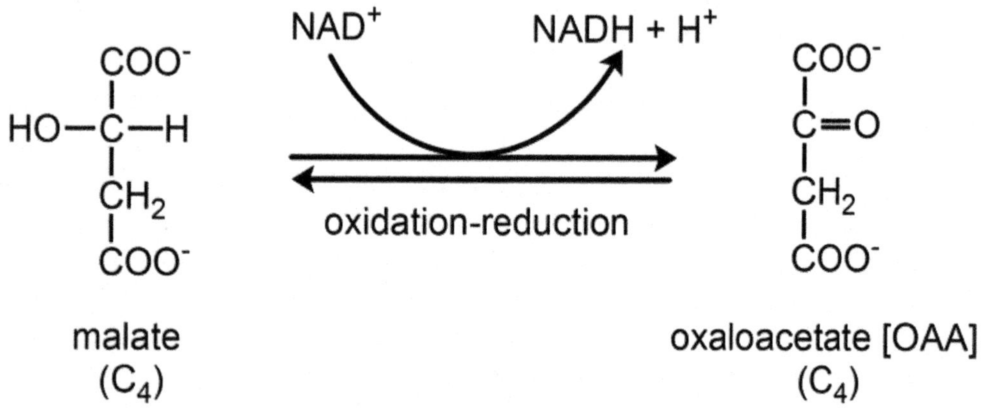

$$NAD^+ \qquad NADH + H^+$$

$$\text{COO}^- \qquad\qquad\qquad \text{COO}^-$$
$$\text{HO}-\text{C}-\text{H} \qquad\qquad \text{C}=\text{O}$$
$$\text{CH}_2 \qquad \text{oxidation-reduction} \qquad \text{CH}_2$$
$$\text{COO}^- \qquad\qquad\qquad \text{COO}^-$$

malate   oxaloacetate [OAA]
(C_4) (C_4)

Enzyme: malate dehydrogenase

Another key determinant in regulating which direction the malate dehydrogenase reaction goes is the ratio of $NADH/NAD^+$ in the mitochondria. When NADH is high in the mitochondria, typically the electron transport chain is slowing down or stopping because plenty of ATP has been made causing the substrates of the ETC (NADH and $FADH_2$) to build up, which inhibits the TCA cycle. These conditions would favor gluconeogenesis, a synthesis pathway, resulting in the reduction of oxaloacetate to malate by malate dehydrogenase for transport to the cytosol. When the cell is doing gluconeogenesis, oxaloacetate is formed from the enzyme pyruvate carboxylase. However, oxaloacetate is not allowed to cross the inner mitochondrial membrane, but malate is. When gluconeogenesis is occurring in a cell, oxaloacetate is quickly reduced to malate for transport to the cytosol. Again, the oxaloacetate concentration is kept low.

Citrate synthase, isocitrate dehydrogenase, and the α-ketoglutarate dehydrogenase complex are the three TCA cycle enzymes that are regulated. While each of these enzymes has several inhibitors and activators, the focus here is on ATP availability as a basic concept of regulation of any metabolic pathway. One should consider if high concentrations of ATP (i.e. a high ATP/ADP ratio) would activate or inhibit the TCA cycle. If the cell has plenty of ATP, the electron transport chain would be inhibited. Thus the mitochondria would have high levels of ATP and NADH, which would inhibit the TCA cycle. NADH inhibits all three of these regulated enzymes, while ATP is an inhibitor of both citrate synthase and isocitrate dehydrogenase. The energy state of the cell also regulates the α-ketoglutarate dehydrogenase complex, as AMP activates the complex.

As mentioned earlier, the TCA Cycle is a provider of intermediates for other biosynthetic pathways. Succinyl CoA provides carbon atoms for porphyrin (heme) synthesis, and α-ketoglutarate and oxaloacetate are intermediates for several amino acid syntheses. The problem is that TCA cycle intermediates must be replenished if any are drawn off for biosynthetic reactions if the cycle needs to continue. The solution is that other reactions, termed anaplerotic reactions (meaning to "fill up"), replenish intermediates. The pyruvate carboxylase reaction can replenish oxaloacetate, and the catabolism of several amino acids form intermediates such as acetyl CoA, fumarate, α-ketoglutarate, and oxaloacetate.

Table 3.2 shows the calculation of net ATP yield from the complete catabolism of a glucose molecule to six molecules of CO_2 (and water), which includes both molecules of pyruvate from glycolysis yielding two molecules of acetyl CoA, via the PDH complex, to turn the TCA cycle two times. To calculate the ATP yield, one needs to consider how the reducing power (NADH and $FADH_2$) produced from glycolysis, the PDH complex and the TCA cycle is used by the electron transport chain to make ATP. NADH donates two electrons to the ETC at Complex I, while $FADH_2$ donates its two electrons at Complex II. The electron movement from NADH to Complexes I, III and IV to ultimately end up on oxygen, which is reduced to water, produces enough electrical energy (proton gradient) to drive the synthesis of about 2.5 ATP (chemical energy). The amount of ATP produced from the reduction of oxygen is termed the P/O ratio. The electron movement from $FADH_2$ to Complexes II, III, and IV to ultimately end up reducing molecular oxygen to water, produces enough electrical energy to drive the synthesis of about 1.5 ATP. So the P/O ratio for NADH is 2.5 ATP per oxygen, and $FADH_2$ is 1.5 ATP per oxygen.

Table 3.2: ATP yield from the complete catabolism of a molecule of glucose.

LOCATION	PATHWAY	YIELD/GLUCOSE	ATP
Cytoplasm	Glycolysis	-2 ATP 4 ATP 2 NADH	-2 +4 +5 [OR +3]* (shuttle dependent)
Mitochondria	PDH Complex	2 NADH	+5
Mitochondria	TCA Cycle	2 GTP 6 NADH 2 FADH$_2$	+2 +15 +3
Total			32 [OR 30]* ATP

*Numbers in brackets indicate lower ATP yield for the glycerol phosphate shuttle, versus the higher number if the malate-aspartate shuttle is used.

In calculating the total yield of ATP from glucose, one must also consider which shuttle is used to transport the electrons from the NADH produced in the cytosol by glyceraldehyde 3-phosphate dehydrogenase in glycolysis. If the malate-aspartate shuttle is used, the electrons from the cytosol end up on a mitochondrial NADH molecule. If the glycerol phosphate shuttle is used, the cytosolic electrons end up on a molecule of $FADH_2$ in the mitochondria, which would yield less ATP. Two molecules of

ATP are also used in the beginning of glycolysis, so these will be subtracted in calculating the net yield.

The complete catabolism of a glucose molecule will yield about 30 to 32 ATP for the cell. In a bomb calorimeter, the combustion of glucose to 6 CO_2 and 6 H_2O would yield approximately 2,870 kJ (686 kcal) of energy released as heat. The hydrolysis of 1 ATP (to ADP + Pi) yields -7.3 kcal/mol. The hydrolysis of 32 ATP yields -234 kcal/mol. The efficiency of the cell to harness the energy released from the oxidation of glucose is about 34% (-234 kcal/mole divided by -686 kcal/mol), which is actually reasonably efficient. To put this number in perspective, most automobile engines are not this efficient in harnessing the energy from the combustion of gasoline.

CHAPTER 4: FATTY ACID OXIDATION AND KETONE BODY SYNTHESIS

Objectives:

1. Define the process of fatty acid oxidation.
    a. Identify the starting and ending products of the pathway, including their structures.
2. Explain the purpose of the pathway of fatty acid oxidation.
    a. Identify all the products of the pathway, the enzymes that produce them, and for what the products can be used.
3. Identify where fatty acid oxidation takes place in the cell, and what tissues can carry out this pathway.
    a. Identify the sources of free fatty acids and how they are transported in the blood.
    b. Explain how acyl CoA is shuttled into the mitochondria and the role of carnitine in the process.
4. Explain how fatty acid oxidation is carried out in the cell.
    a. Describe the four repeated steps of fatty acid oxidation, and identify the enzymes and cofactors involved in these steps.
    b. Calculate the number of cycles needed to oxidize fatty acids of even- and odd-numbered chain lengths, and the total number of products produced (i.e. the number of acetyl CoA, propionyl CoA, $FADH_2$, and NADH produced for the complete oxidation of the fatty acid in question).
5. Explain when fatty acid oxidation takes place.
    a. Identify the regulatory enzymes of fatty acid oxidation; identify what is the primary regulator of CAT I and how hormones regulate fatty acid oxidation.
6. Define the process of ketone body synthesis.
    a. Identify the starting and ending products of the pathway, including their structures.
7. Explain the purpose of the pathway of ketone body synthesis.
    a. Identify all the products of the pathway, the enzymes that produce them, and for what the products can be used.
8. Identify where ketone body synthesis takes place in the cell, and what tissue(s) can carry out this pathway.

9. Explain how fatty acid oxidation is carried out in the cell, and how ketone bodies are utilized by other tissues.

    a. Describe the steps of ketone body synthesis, and explain the fates of the 3 ketone bodies produced.

10. Explain when ketone body synthesis takes place (i.e. under what conditions are ketone bodies produced).

    a. Explain the regulation by acetyl CoA concentrations that coordinate fatty acid oxidation, ketone body synthesis, and gluconeogenesis.

    b. Explain why starvation increases ketone body production.

OVERVIEW OF LIPID METABOLISM

Lipids are an important source of fuel for the body. One pound of fat (triacylglycerols) will yield about 4,000 kcal. One pound of glycogen, the storage form of glucose, will yield about 400 kcal. If one understands the basic recipe of metabolism, this makes sense. The more oxidation steps that must be done to oxidize carbons to carboxylic acids, the more $FADH_2$ and NADH are produced, which is used by the electron transport chain for the production of ATP. A 16-carbon fatty acid (i.e. palmitate) has 15 carbons that are at the level of an alkane, and one carbon already at the level of a carboxylic acid. To oxidize all 15 of these carbons up to carboxylic acids, so they can be clipped off as CO_2 to burn them off, will produce a lot of $FADH_2$ and NADH for ultimate ATP production. Glucose, on the other hand, is only six carbons. Of these 6 carbons, five of them are at the level of an alcohol and one carbon is at the level of an aldehyde. Glucose has less carbons, and they are already more oxidized than a fatty acid. Therefore, the cell has to do less oxidation reactions to oxidize these carbons to carboxylic acids, and less $FADH_2$ and NADH is produced. Fatty acids, then, are the body's major storage form of energy, and are stored as triacylglycerols (TAG).

Another benefit to storing triacylglycerols over glycogen is that triacylglycerols (a.k.a. triglycerides or fats) are hydrophobic, meaning they do not like water. A triacylglycerol molecule (i.e. fat) consists of three fatty acids linked through ester bonds to glycerol, as shown in **Figure 4.1**. Glycogen, though, is hydrophilic and has water associated with it. By storing more fuel as triacylglycerols, than as glycogen, the body will not have excess weight due to water associated with glycogen.

The tissues of the body must always have ready access to a fuel source that is circulating through the blood, which the author terms "fast food." Lipids, though, are not our "fast food" or readily available circulating fuel source. The hydrophobicity of lipids makes them a great storage form of fuel, but not a circulating fuel source. Because lipids are hydrophobic, they are not easily transported in the blood, which largely consists of water. Maintaining a circulating supply of lipids in the blood is more difficult, as lipids like triacylglycerols and cholesterols must be packaged in special vesicles called lipoprotein particles (i.e. chylomicrons, VLDLs, LDLs, and HDLs). Individual fatty acids, themselves, must be attached to a carrier protein, albumin, for transport through the blood.

Thus, fat accounts for most of our stored energy, but it is not the body's primary "circulating fuel" because it hates water. Glucose does like water, as it is hydrophilic and water-soluble. A cell cannot get as much energy from a molecule of glucose, but it is easier to circulate in the blood. Therefore, glucose serves as the primary water-soluble fuel source that is readily available (i.e. "fast food") for use by tissues. Ketone bodies, which are water-soluble derivatives of fatty acids, are a second major "circulating fuel" that will be also be discussed in this chapter.

Figure 4.1: Basic structure of a triacylglycerol and the structures of the common glycerophospholipids

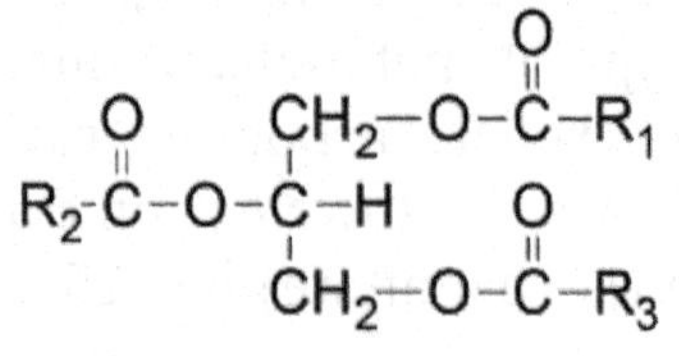

Triacylglycerol

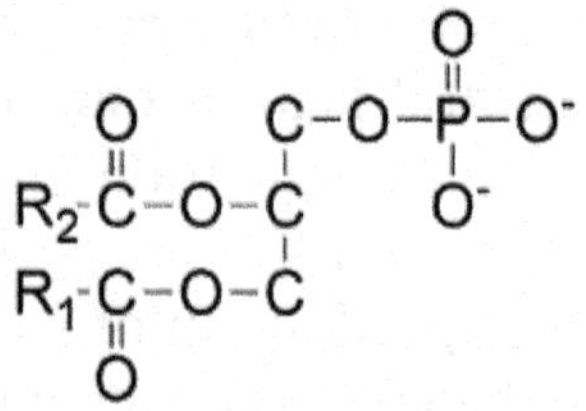

Phosphatidate
(Phosphatidic acid, when protonated)

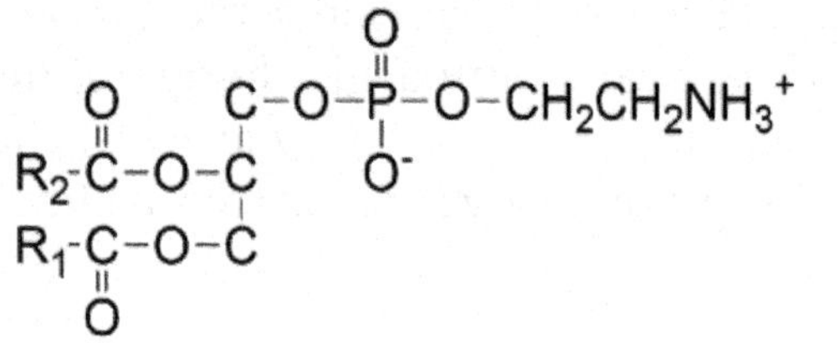

Phosphatidylethanolamine

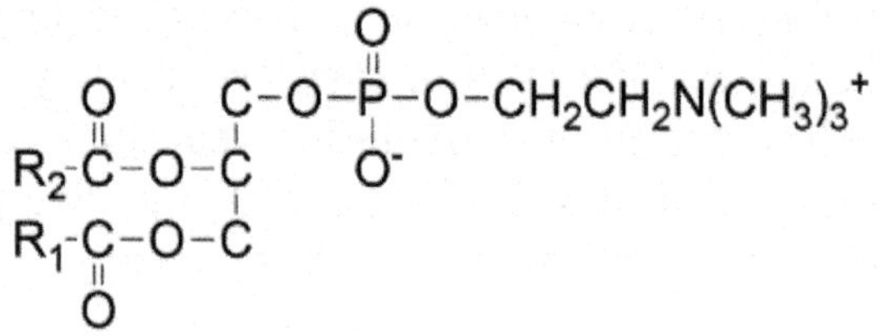

Phosphatidylcholine
(a.k.a. lecithin)

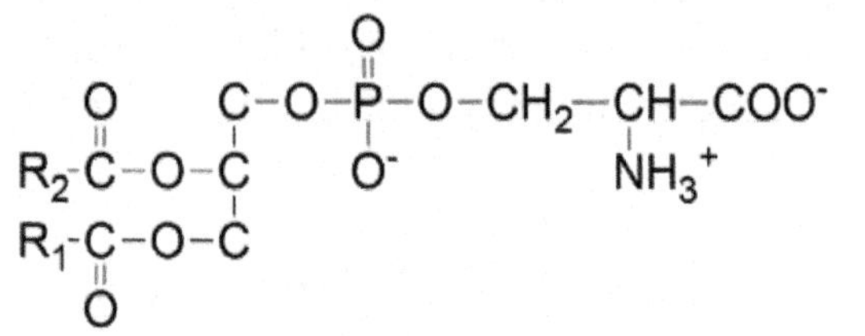

Phosphatidylserine

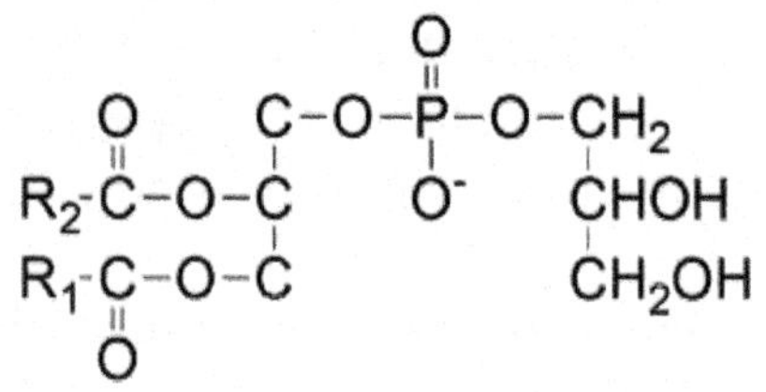

Phosphatidylglycerol

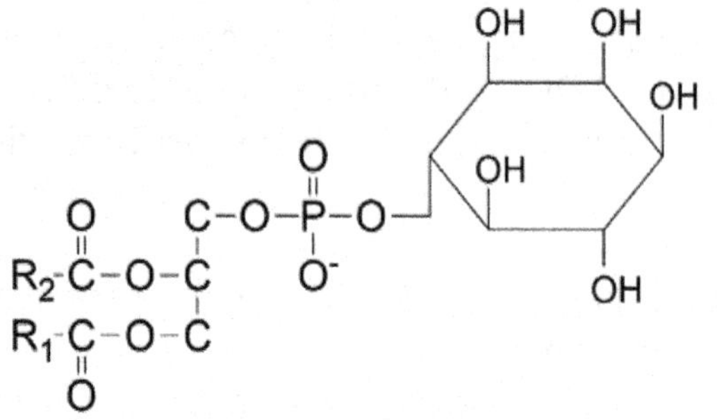

Phosphatidylinositol

R = hydrocarbon portion of fatty acids, may be saturated or unsaturated

Lipids are also important structural components of biological membranes. These lipids include phospholipids (i.e. glycerophospholipids) shown in **Figure 4.1**, sphingolipids, glycolipids, and cholesterol. Membranes are lipid bilayers. Membranes form hydrophobic barriers and are responsible for compartmentation of cells. Lipids that reside in membranes must be amphipathic, meaning they have a hydrophilic (polar) portion and a hydrophobic (nonpolar) portion of the molecule. The hydrophilic region can interact with water, and the hydrophobic portion will form the hydrophobic center of a membrane. Reciprocal pathways often take place in separate compartments of a cell, or at least some portion of one of the pathways occurs in a different compartment. For instance, many catabolic pathways are in the mitochondria, while synthetic pathways are often in the cytosol (though there are exceptions in both compartments). Some lipid components of membranes play important roles in signal transduction pathways, as well as lipids that serve as hormones (i.e. steroid hormones and the eicosanoid hormones, derived from arachidonic acid shown in **Table 4.1**).

Table 4.1: Fatty Acids of Importance to Humans

Numerical symbol	Structure	Trivial name	Systematic name
16:0	CH_3-$(CH_2)_{14}$-COOH	Palmitic	Hexadecanoic
18:2(9,12)	CH_3-$(CH_2)_3$-$(CH_2$-$CH=CH)_2$-$(CH_2)_7$-COOH	Linoleic	*cis,cis*9,12-Octadecatrienoic
18:3(9,12,15)	CH_3-$(CH_2$-$CH=CH)_3$-$(CH_2)_7$-COOH	Linolenic	*cis,cis,cis*-9,12,15-Octadecatrienoic
20:4(5,8,11,14)	CH_3-$(CH_2)_3$-$(CH_2$-$CH=CH)_4$-$(CH_2)_3$-COOH	Arachidonic	*cis,cis,cis,cis*-5,8,11,14-Icosatetraenoic

Other lipids must be obtained in the diet. There are four lipid-soluble vitamins (vitamins A, D, E, and K) which are important to obtain in the diet, as they carry out important biological functions, of which a few functions are described here. Vitamin A derivatives are important visual pigments and hormones. Vitamin A is commonly found in fish liver oils, liver, eggs, whole milk and butter. The yellow vegetables, such as carrots and sweet potatoes, provide β-carotene that can also be converted to vitamin A. Vitamin D derivatives are important hormones for regulation of calcium levels, which is important for bone formation. Vitamin D_3 is formed in skin from a cholesterol derivative using ultraviolet (UV) rays of sunlight. Not all people get sufficient amounts naturally, so similar vitamin D derivatives are added to milk and juice products, as well. Vitamin E derivatives serve as important antioxidants and vitamin K derivatives are important in the blood clotting cascade. Vitamin E is abundant in wheat germ, and can also be obtained from eggs and vegetable oils. Forms of vitamin K are obtained from green leafy vegetables and some intestinal bacteria.

Linoleic and linolenic acids are two essential fatty acids for humans (see **Table 4.1**). These two fatty acids must be obtained in the diet, as will be discussed further. These are the omega-6 (ω-6) and omega-3 (ω-3) fatty acids, one commonly hears about regarding dietary supplements. Recall that the "omega" carbon is the methyl end carbon of a fatty acid (see **Figure 1.1**). In counting in from the methyl end the molecule, an omega-6 fatty acid will have its first double bond six carbons in; while an omega-3 fatty acid has its first double bond three carbons in from the methyl end of the molecule.

While the synthesis of complex lipid structures (i.e. triacylglycerols, phospholipids, lipid hormones, etc.) will not be covered in this textbook, understanding what fatty acids are used for in the cell is important. Membrane lipids (i.e. phospholipids, sphingolipids, and glycolipids), triacylglycerols, and lipoproteins all have fatty acids as components. Thus, knowing the catabolism of what molecules serve as the source of fatty acids for fatty acid oxidation, as well as the possible fates of a newly synthesized fatty acid is an important level of understanding for the lipid pathways covered in this text. A cell will not, though, synthesize a new fatty acid only to turn around and break it down in fatty acid oxidation, as that would be a futile cycle. Fatty acid oxidation and fatty acid synthesis, as reciprocal pathways, are regulated such that both of these pathways are not on at the same time in the same cell.

FATTY ACID OXIDATION (a.k.a. β-oxidation or FA degradation)

The name of this pathway is its definition (what?). Fatty acid oxidation, also known as β-oxidation of fatty acids, is the breakdown or catabolism of fatty acids, via oxidation at the β-carbon, to form acetyl CoA. In this pathway, the starting material is a fatty acid in which carbon #3 (the β-carbon) is at the level of an alkane. The β-carbon of the fatty acid will need to be oxidized to a ketone, prior to clipping off a molecule of acetyl CoA.

The purpose (why?) of β-oxidation of fatty acids is to produce reducing power in the form of $FADH_2$ and NADH that will donate their electrons directly to the electron transport chain for ATP production. The acetyl CoA can be sent into the TCA cycle to further catabolize the 2 carbon "acetyl" unit to carbon dioxide (CO_2) and produce more reducing power to be used for ATP production. In the liver, the acetyl CoA can also be used for ketone body production.

This pathway takes place (where?) in the mitochondrial matrix. However, the free fatty acids are in the cytosol and the cell needs to move them into the matrix. Therefore, there is a transport step needed for this pathway. Most tissues can take up fatty acids circulating in the blood for fuel, except for mature red blood cells (erythrocytes) and the brain. Erythrocytes cannot use fatty acids because they lack mitochondria. The brain cannot import fatty acids from the blood because fatty acids cannot cross the blood-brain barrier. However, neurons can catabolize fatty acids from their own cellular membrane turn-over, etc.

The overview of the pathway of β-oxidation of fatty acids is shown in **Figure 4.2**. For learning the process (how?) of fatty acid oxidation, one needs to know the sources of fatty acids and how they are transported into the mitochondrial matrix. The four repeated steps of β-oxidation, though, should make sense based on one's understanding of the oxidation states flow chart (**Figure 1.7**) for the series of reactions required to put a keto group on a carbon. In fact, exercise #4 at the end of the chapter 1 (the oxidation states chapter) required one to put in order the correct sequence of molecules for the first three reactions of β-oxidation based on their structures, and name the enzymes for these reactions.

Figure 4.2: Overview of β-oxidation of fatty acids

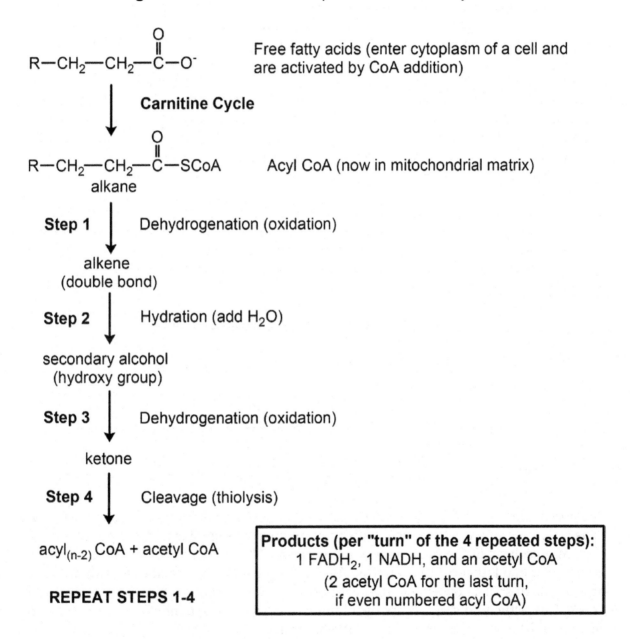

The sources of the fatty acids include dietary fats, stored body fat (i.e. triacylglycerols in adipose cells), and membrane lipid turnover. Membranes are constantly be damaged and repaired, or synthesized. Thus the degradation of membrane components such as phospholipids, sphingolipids or glycolipids can provide fatty acids for fatty acid oxidation.

Lipases are enzymes that cleave components from the complex lipids such as phospholipids or triacylglycerols. There are specific types of lipases that act on the specific classes of complex lipids. Hormone-sensitive lipase is a hormonally controlled lipase that clips fatty acids off stored triacylglycerol molecules. Several types of phospholipases cleave the fatty acids and the headgroups from the various phospholipids. The pancreas secretes lipases in the digestion of various dietary lipids.

As lipids are hydrophobic, the transport of lipids through the blood is a complex process. The larger complex lipids, like triacylglycerols and cholesterol esters, are transported in the blood in vesicles called lipoprotein particles, which has a monolayer of phospholipids and specific proteins. Individual fatty acid molecules must also be transported in the blood using a carrier. Albumin, a protein, is the carrier of individual fatty acids through the blood.

Individual or "free" fatty acids are not components of membranes, and they must always be attached to a carrier molecule inside or outside of a cell. Free fatty acids act as detergents and will break up membranes causing a cell to lyse. As fatty acids are brought into a cell or synthesized *de novo*, they are quickly attached to a carrier molecule, usually coenzyme A.

Figure 4.3: Activation of a free fatty acid

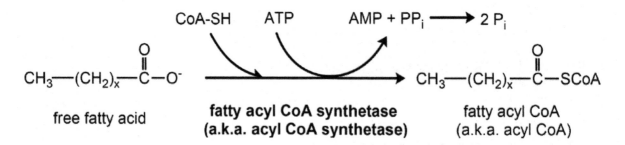

The attachment of a fatty acid to a cellular carrier requires an input of energy, referred to as activation of a free fatty acid. This input of energy is similar to the input of energy used in glycolysis in the beginning of the pathway. The activation of a fatty acid is the attachment of a fatty acid to coenzyme A (CoA) using ATP, as shown in **Figure 4.3**. The product of this reaction is a "fatty acyl-CoA," or more simply referred to as an "acyl CoA." This activation step occurs by a family of isozymes (depending on the fatty acid chain length) in the outer mitochondrial membrane.

The name of the family of isozymes for this step indicates the reaction they carry out. An enzyme that synthesizes bonds between two molecules to form larger products is called either a *synthase* or a *synthetase*. A synthase does not require energy, while a synthetase does require energy. Both synthases and synthetases are named for the product of the reaction. In this reaction ATP is used to attach a fatty acid to the free sulfhydryl group of coenzyme A forming a thioester bond between the two molecules. The product of the reaction is a fatty acyl CoA (a.k.a. acyl CoA). Therefore the name of the family of enzymes that catalyzes this reaction is **fatty acyl CoA synthetase**, or simply **acyl CoA synthetase**. The various isozymes of the acyl Co synthetases work on fatty acids that are of short, intermediate, or long carbon chains.

In the reaction, two phosphates of ATP are cleaved off to form AMP plus a molecule called pyrophosphate (PP_i). Pyrophosphate is immediately cleaved by an enzyme called pyrophosphatase to form two inorganic phosphate groups. The cleavage of pyrophosphate drives the reaction forward and makes this reaction irreversible. This cleavage of two high energy phosphate bonds is the equivalent of 2 ATP forming 2 ADP molecules, which will become important when calculating ATP yields from the complete catabolism of a fatty acid.

At this point the fatty acid is in the cytosol of the cell safely attached to coenzyme A. This acyl CoA does not have to be transported into the mitochondrial matrix for further catabolism. It could be used for membrane lipids, if the cell needs to repair membranes or synthesize new membranes; for storage on a triacylglycerol molecule; for the formation of a lipoprotein, etc. The cell does not have to transport the acyl CoA into the mitochondria. If the cell does need to catabolize the fatty acid further via β-oxidation, the acyl CoA does need to be transported into the mitochondrial matrix, as will be described next.

The fatty acid was activated to an acyl CoA on the outer mitochondrial membrane, and the cell now needs to get it into the mitochondrial matrix. The carnitine cycle is the process by which the cell transports the acyl CoA molecules into the mitochondrial matrix for β-oxidation. Recall that the inner mitochondrial membrane is very impermeable. Special transporters are required to move molecules across the inner mitochondrial membrane. The process of moving the fatty acid into matrix requires two enzymes and a transporter. The two enzymes are carnitine acyltransferase I (CAT I) and carnitine acyltransferase II (CAT II), see **Figure 4.4**. CAT I is a regulated enzyme located in the outer mitochondrial membrane. CAT I exchanges the coenzyme A on an acyl CoA for carnitine to form acyl-carnitine. The formation of the acyl carnitine by CAT I commits the fatty acid for movement into the mitochondria for further catabolism.

The transporter is called the acyl-carnitine/carnitine translocase (or transporter). When a transporter in the inner mitochondrial membrane "opens," it typically lets a molecule into the matrix and lets something out. In this case, the translocase transports acyl-carnitine into the matrix and "free" carnitine is transported out. Once the acyl-carnitine is in the matrix, CAT II (located in the inner mitochondrial membrane) clips the carnitine molecule off and attaches the fatty acid back onto a coenzyme A molecule—reforming an acyl CoA that is now located in the mitochondrial matrix for catabolism by the β-oxidation pathway. CAT II is not regulated.

Carnitine can be obtained from dietary sources, primarily in meat. Carnitine can also be synthesized from lysine and methionine, but only in the liver and kidneys. Other tissues, especially the heart and skeletal muscles depend on carnitine from endogenous synthesis in the liver and kidneys or from the diet. Carnitine from either of these sources must be circulated in the blood for uptake by these tissues. Skeletal muscle, of particular note, contains over 95% of all of the carnitine in the body. Strict vegetarians and vegans may need to ensure they are getting plenty of carnitine from alternative dietary sources.

Figure 4.4: The carnitine shuttle

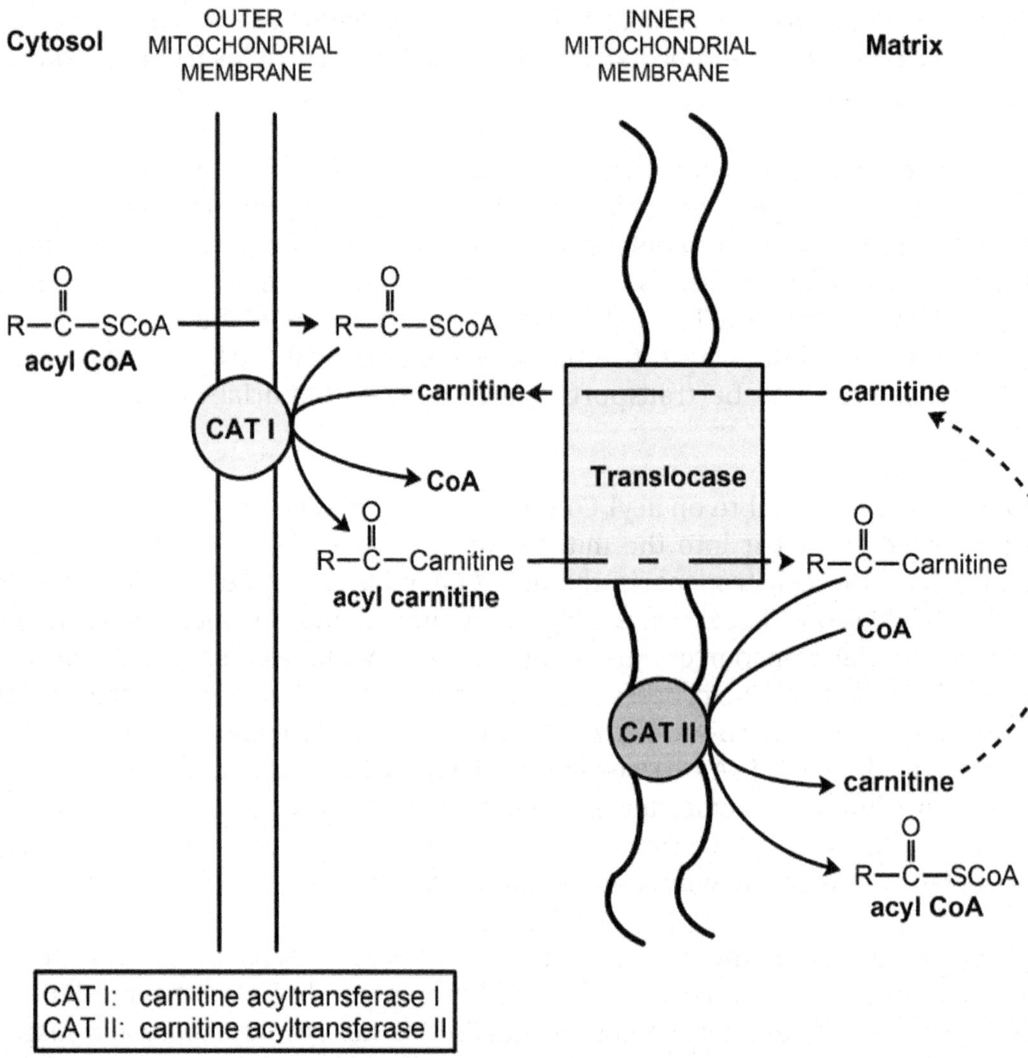

CAT I: carnitine acyltransferase I
CAT II: carnitine acyltransferase II

Exercise #4 at the end of the oxidation states chapter is putting in order the first three steps of the four repeated steps of fatty acid oxidation. For fatty acid oxidation a keto group needs to be put on a carbon that is initially at the level of an alkane. This pathway proceeds from the top of oxidation states flow chart down to the ketone group (shown in **Figure 1.7**). This is the exact same sequence of three reactions seen in the TCA cycle to go from succinate to oxaloacetate. In exercise #4, the molecules were named using the first letter of their molecular name. The goal of β-oxidation of fatty acids is to produce acetyl CoA and reducing power in the form of FADH$_2$ and NADH. The starting material shown in **Figure 4.5**, is a fatty acyl CoA—specifically palmitoyl CoA, a 16-carbon fatty acid attached to coenzyme A. Palmitate is one of the more common fatty acids in humans. If the cell simply clipped off the first two carbons of the fatty acid attached to the coenzyme A, a molecule of acetyl CoA would be produced. However, the other product would be a hydrocarbon, a molecule with only carbons and hydrogens. Hydrocarbons are very hydrophobic and un-reactive. A cell would not be able to do anything with a hydrocarbon product. Therefore, the four-step reaction sequence of the pathway of β-oxidation of fatty acids is set up to yield a molecule of acetyl CoA and a fatty acyl CoA molecule that is two carbons shorter than the acyl CoA used in the first reaction. The shorter fatty acid can then continue to be catabolized in subsequent rounds of these 4 steps. The sequence of the four repeated steps of β-oxidation of fatty acids is shown in **Figure 4.5**.

The name "β-oxidation of fatty acids" indicates exactly what happens in this pathway. The β-carbon (i.e. carbon #3) of the fatty acid is oxidized. Specifically the β-carbon is oxidized to a keto group. In **Figure 4.5**, carbon #3, the β-carbon is at the level of an alkane in palmitoyl CoA (or any acyl CoA). Following the oxidation states flow chart (**Figure 1.7**), an alkane can be oxidized to a keto group by first oxidizing to an alkene, then hydration to a secondary alcohol, followed by oxidation to a keto group. The first three steps of β-oxidation are those exact three steps.

In step #1, the acyl-CoA (palmitoyl CoA for this example) is oxidized to an enoyl CoA. Enoyl CoA is the generic name for any fatty acid containing a double bond (i.e. an unsaturated fatty acid). To be more specific, the double bond introduced in this step is a *trans* double bond, as opposed to the normal *cis* double bonds that are introduced into unsaturated fatty acids that will be incorporated into membrane lipids for structural reasons. The *cis* double bonds produce "kinks" in the fatty acid chains, preventing them from packing together tightly and allowing membranes to be more fluid. In this reaction, though, the *trans* configuration of the double bond is fine because the double bond will be removed in the next step. Recall from the oxidation states chapter that when oxidizing from an alkane to an alkene, FAD is the coenzyme used for the coupled reduction reaction, as shown in **Figure 4.5**.

Enzymes that carry out oxidation-reduction reactions using NAD$^+$ or FAD are called *dehydrogenases*. Dehydrogenases are named for the more reduced molecule. Therefore the name of the enzyme for reaction #1 is ***fatty acyl CoA dehydrogenase***, or more simply ***acyl CoA dehydrogenase***. In the mitochondria, there is a family of different acyl

CoA dehydrogenases (i.e. isozymes) that that have distinct, yet overlapping, specificities for fatty acids of particular chain lengths. For example, long-chain acyl CoA dehydrogenase (LCAD) works on fatty acids of about 12 to 18 carbons, medium-chain acyl CoA dehydrogenase (MCAD) works on fatty acids of about 4 to 14 carbons, while short-chain acyl CoA dehydrogenase (SCAD) acts on fatty acids of about 4 to 8 carbons.

Figure 4.5: The four repeated steps of β-oxidation

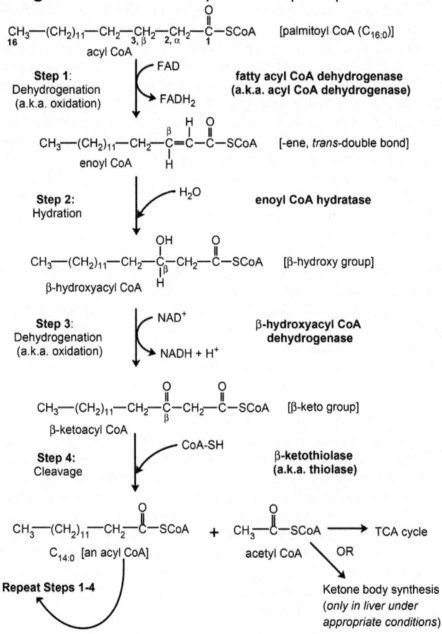

In step #2, water is added across the double bond of the enoyl CoA such that the hydroxy group is placed on the β-carbon (carbon #3) forming a secondary alcohol group. The product of this reaction is called β-hydroxyacyl CoA (or 3-hydroxyacyl CoA). This reaction is adding water to the molecule, so the enzyme is called a *hydratase*. The enzyme is named after the molecule that is accepting the water molecule, enoyl CoA. Thus, the enzyme is called **enoyl CoA hydratase**.

In step #3, the secondary alcohol of β-hydroxyacyl CoA is oxidized to a ketone forming β-ketoacyl CoA. This is an oxidation reaction, so a reduction reaction must simultaneously occur. NAD^+ is reduced to $NADH + H^+$, as is typical for oxidations of alcohols to ketones. Enzymes that carry out oxidation-reduction reactions using NAD^+ or FAD are called *dehydrogenases*. Dehydrogenases are named for the more reduced molecule, which is β-hydroxyacyl CoA. The enzyme that catalyzes reaction #3 is thus named **β-hydroxyacyl CoA dehydrogenase**.

At this point a keto group is now on the β-carbon (carbon #3) of a fatty acid. Hopefully, the three reactions needed to accomplish this make sense in the context of the oxidation states flow chart (or "basic recipe of metabolism"). In step #4, a molecule of acetyl CoA is cleaved off using another molecule of coenzyme A to produce a 2-carbon shorter acyl CoA (a 14-carbon fatty acyl CoA, as shown in **Figure 4.5**). The enzyme that catalyzes this reaction is called **β-ketothiolase** (or just **thiolase**). By putting the keto group on the β-position of the fatty acid, a molecule of coenzyme A with is free sulfhydryl (or thiol) group is now used to cleave the bond (i.e. "thiolase") between carbons 2 and 3 and is attached to the keto carbon producing a new shorter fatty acyl CoA, along with a molecule of acetyl CoA. The 14-carbon fatty acid can continue to be catabolized through subsequent rounds of these 4 steps of β-oxidation.

For calculating how much ATP can be produced from the catabolism of a fatty acid, one first needs to figure out how many acetyl CoA molecules can be formed from the catabolism of a fatty acid and how many "cycles" of these four repeated steps are needed to make those molecules of acetyl CoA. If the starting fatty acid has an even number of carbons, just divide the number by 2 (because the acetyl unit is 2 carbons). For the 16-carbon fatty acid shown in **Figure 4.5**, a total of 8 acetyl CoA molecules can be produced. Seven cycles of the four repeated steps are needed to produce those 8 acetyl CoA molecules because the last round is starting with a 4-carbon fatty acid, which forms the last 2 acetyl CoA molecules when it is cut in half by the thiolase. Those 7 cycles of the four repeated steps will also yield 7 $FADH_2$ molecules and 7 NADH molecules. Since this pathway occurs in the mitochondrial matrix, the $FADH_2$ and NADH molecules can deliver their electrons directly to the electron transport chain. The 8 acetyl CoA molecules will now "turn" the TCA cycle 8 times, producing even more reducing power and some GTP, while completely catabolizing the fatty acids to CO_2.

Table 4.2 shows the net energy (ATP) yield from the complete oxidation of palmitoyl CoA, the 16-carbon saturated fatty acid, to 16 molecules of CO_2. Recall that an NADH yields about 2.5 ATP, and an $FADH_2$ yields about 1.5 ATP from the electron transport chain. As one can see from the table, about 106 ATP can be produced from the catabolism of a fatty acid, which is much more than a molecule of glucose (30 to 32 ATP). The catabolism of a fatty acid produces much more reducing power (NADH and $FADH_2$) formed during the oxidation of the carbons from the level of an alkane to a ketone in the four repeated steps, and then to carboxylic acids in the TCA cycle.

Table 4.2: Net energy (ATP) yield from the complete catabolism of palmitoyl CoA (C_{16})

Products of β-oxidation	From TCA cycle		ATP yield
8 acetyl CoA	(8 x) 3 NADH	(x 2.5)	60
	(8 x) 1 $FADH_2$	(x 1.5)	12
	(8 x) 1 GTP	(x 1)	8
7 $FADH_2$	(x 1.5)		10.5
7 NADH	(x 2.5)		17.5
			108
*2 high energy PO_4^{2-} bonds broken during activation stage (ATP to AMP + PP_i; PP_i to $2P_i$)			- 2
			106 ATP (Net yield)

The body contains more than just 16-carbon saturated fatty acids, both obtained in the diet and from *de novo* synthesis. There are odd-numbered carbon chain fatty acids, branched chain fatty acids, and unsaturated fatty acids. Unsaturated fatty acids are fatty acids that have one or more double bonds, usually in the *cis* configuration. *Cis* double bonds introduce a structural change in the hydrocarbon portion of the fatty acid preventing these types of fatty acids, particularly on membrane lipids, from packing together as tightly and allowing for membrane fluidity.

The enoyl CoA hydratase (for reaction #2) can only hydrate an enoyl CoA that has a *trans* double bond between carbons #2 and #3. Often during rounds of the four repeated steps of β-oxidation of an unsaturated fatty acid a *cis* double bond is encountered either between carbons #2 and #3 or between carbons #3 and #4. In either of these cases, the enzyme **enoyl CoA isomerase** isomerizes the double bond to a *trans* double bond, and if necessary moves it between carbons #2 and #3. An $FADH_2$ molecule will not be formed for that round of repeated steps because the molecule already has a double bond (i.e. enoyl CoA isomerase catalyzes the first step of that round, rather than the acyl CoA dehydrogenase enzyme).

Figure 4.6: Conversion of propionyl CoA, from β-oxidation of odd-numbered carbon fatty acids, to succinyl CoA for complete oxidation by the TCA cycle.

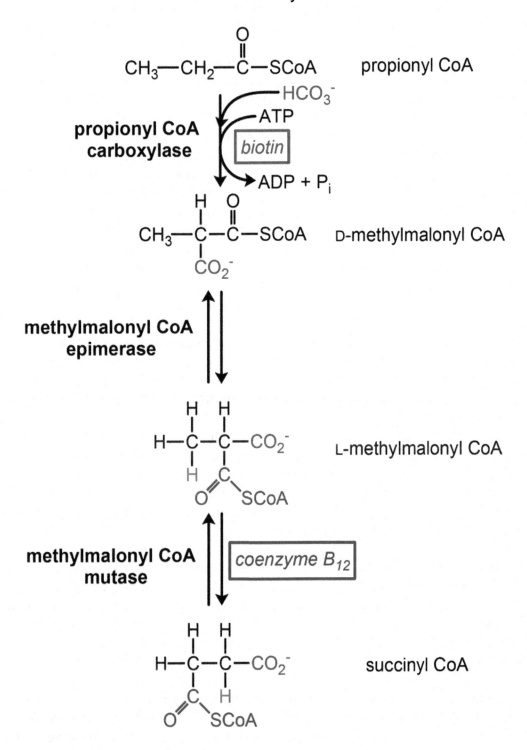

For fatty acids that have an odd-numbered carbon chain length (i.e. a 17-carbon length fatty acid), the "last" round of 4 repeated steps starts with a 5-carbon long fatty acid. In the thiolase step, an acetyl CoA molecule is produced along with a 3-carbon fatty acyl CoA called propionyl CoA. The cell still needs to further catabolize this molecule by getting it into the TCA cycle. The propionyl CoA is converted to succinyl CoA in three reactions, as shown in **Figure 4.6**. The first enzymatic reaction requires ATP and CO_2 (from bicarbonate, HCO_3^-), to carboxylate the propionyl CoA to a 4-carbon molecule called D-methylmalonyl CoA. The enzyme that catalyzes this reaction is ***propionyl CoA carboxylase***, and requires biotin and carries out a similar mechanism as other carboxylases (i.e. pyruvate carboxylase and acetyl CoA carboxylase). The second reaction is catalyzed by ***methylmalonyl CoA epimerase***, which isomerizes D-methylmalonyl CoA to L-methylmalonyl CoA. The third reaction is catalyzed by ***methylmalonyl CoA mutase***, and requires a coenzyme form of Vitamin B_{12}. This reaction is unusual in that a hydrogen and the carbonyl CoA group on adjacent carbons exchange positions to form succinyl CoA, which can then enter the TCA cycle. The propionyl CoA molecule will not yield as much GTP and reducing power as an acetyl CoA molecule because it enters the TCA cycle further into the cycle. Note that the formation of succinyl CoA from propionyl CoA is the only gluconeogenic precursor derived from the catabolism of fatty acids because succinyl CoA enters the TCA cycle after the points where the two molecules of CO_2 are formed.

There are also other types of fatty acid catabolic processes located in other organelles, which are briefly described here. In peroxisomes, β-oxidation works primarily on very-long carbon chain length fatty acids (i.e. hexacosanoic acid, a $C_{26:0}$) and branched chain fatty acids such as phytanic acid and pristanic acid. Branched chain fatty acids typically have a methyl group in the β-carbon position, which does not allow for oxidation of the β-carbon. Therefore, catabolism of the branched chain fatty acids in the peroxisomes uses a process called α-oxidation. In α-oxidation, the branched fatty acid is oxidized to a hydroxyl group on the α-carbon and then shortened by one carbon by decarboxylation forming an aldehyde, which is subsequently oxidized to a carboxylic acid. Peroxisomes catabolize fatty acids to shorter carbon-chain lengths, which are then transported to the mitochondrial matrix for complete oxidation.

Another process for fatty acid catabolism is ω-oxidation, which is oxidation of the ω-carbon (the methyl end). This type of fatty acid catabolism occurs in the endoplasmic reticulum and is normally a relatively minor pathway of fatty acid catabolism in humans (and other mammals). However, fatty acid catabolism by ω-oxidation is up-regulated in individuals with a defect in an enzyme of β-oxidation, or in those who have a carnitine deficiency.

There are several enzymes involved in the regulation of β-oxidation of fatty acids, including the sources and transport of fatty acids to the matrix. Hormone-sensitive lipase, which is an important enzyme in clipping off fatty acids from triacylglycerols in adipose tissue, is hormonally regulated. Insulin (high blood sugar indicator) and glucagon (low blood sugar) are two important hormones that regulate this lipase.

Glucagon stimulates hormone-sensitive lipase in adipose tissue because, as will be covered next, the fatty acids will be transported via albumin to the liver (one of the main target tissues of glucagon) and be used for ketone body synthesis. In the fed state (insulin predominates) excess nutrients are stored as fat (triacylglycerols). When insulin is the predominant hormone, the hormone-sensitive lipases are inhibited because fatty acid synthesis and triacylglycerol synthesis are occurring in the cells to store these nutrients.

The key regulation, though, of β-oxidation of fatty acids occurs at the point of transport into the mitochondrial matrix. Fatty acids, as well as being an important fuel source, are also structures of membrane lipids, lipoproteins, etc. Once a fatty acid is transported into the mitochondrial matrix, the fatty acid is essentially committed to the oxidative fate (i.e. catabolism). As mentioned previously, carnitine acyltransferase I (CAT I) is a regulated enzyme. CAT I is inhibited by high concentrations of malonyl CoA, which is a substrate for fatty acid synthesis. The transport of fatty acids into the mitochondria matrix (of which the first step is carried out by CAT I) will be inhibited if fatty acid synthesis is occurring in the cell. The cell does not want to expend energy synthesizing a fatty acid, only to turn around and break it down by β-oxidation. That would be a futile cycle. Therefore these reciprocal pathways are not on at the same time in the same cell, and there are specific regulators to ensure that does not happen.

Two of the enzymatic steps of β-oxidation are also regulated: β-hydroxyacyl CoA dehydrogenase and β-ketothiolase. The ratio of [NADH]/[NAD⁺] regulates β-hydroxyacyl CoA dehydrogenase. When this ratio is high, NADH predominates indicating the cell has plenty of energy (i.e. the electron transport chain is inhibited due to plenty of ATP), which inhibits this enzyme. High concentrations of acetyl CoA inhibits β-ketothiolase, which is another indicator of sufficient energy in the cell.

KETONE BODY SYNTHESIS

Ketone body synthesis (what?) is the synthesis of water-soluble derivatives of lipids. The cell catabolizes fatty acids (via β-oxidation) to form acetyl CoA, which will be used to form water-soluble derivatives called ketone bodies. Of the three molecules referred to as ketone bodies, only two of them actually have a keto group, as will be discussed further.

The purpose of the production of ketone bodies (why?) is that they are used in proportion to their blood concentration by extra hepatic tissues. Skeletal and cardiac muscle use them, and the renal cortex has a preference for them. During starvation or diabetic conditions, ketone bodies become a major fuel source for the brain. Since the fatty acids cannot cross the blood-brain barrier, ketone bodies (as water-soluble derivatives of fatty acids) can cross the blood-brain barrier. The brain prefers glucose over ketone bodies, which is one reason why maintaining glucose in the blood is a metabolic priority. The brain will use ketone bodies, but it usually requires about 48 hours of glucose starvation before the brain will begin to use them. Note that mature red blood cells cannot use ketone bodies. Cells that utilize ketone bodies convert them back to two molecules of acetyl CoA in the mitochondria. Since mature red blood cells do not have mitochondria, they cannot use ketone bodies as a fuel source.

Ketone body synthesis takes place (where?) in the liver mitochondrial matrix. Only the liver can do ketone body synthesis. While the liver synthesizes the ketone bodies, it cannot use them because it lacks the enzyme needed to convert acetoacetate to acetoacetyl CoA. The lack of this enzyme prevents the liver from doing a futile cycle of synthesis and breakdown of ketone bodies.

In ketone body synthesis (how?), all of the carbons of the ketone bodies come from molecules of acetyl CoA. While ketone bodies are 3 or 4 carbons, their synthesis proceeds through a six-carbon activated intermediate, 3-hydroxy-3-methylglutaryl CoA (HMG-CoA). There are three ketone bodies, and **Figure 4.7** shows the pathway of ketone body synthesis.

The pathway is three to four steps, depending on the ketone body produced. Reaction #1 starts with the condensation of two molecules of acetyl CoA and **β-ketothiolase** (the same "enzyme #4" of β-oxidation) carries out the reverse reaction to produce acetoacetyl CoA. The name "acetoacetyl CoA" indicates its structure: two acetate molecules connected together end to end attached to coenzyme A.

The pathway goes through a 6-carbon intermediate using a third acetyl CoA molecule. In reaction #2, this third molecule of acetyl CoA is condensed at its methyl carbon to carbon #3 of acetoacetyl CoA. The removal of the coenzyme A from this third molecule of acetyl CoA drives the reaction forward to form the six-carbon product 3-hydroxy-3-methylglutaryl CoA (HMG-CoA). The full name of the molecule indicates its structure. The "glut" indicates a 5 carbon structure, which is similar to the 5 carbon "straight chain" portion of citrate. Draw 5 carbons with a carboxylic acid group at each end, with $-CH_2$ groups on carbons 2 and 4. The "3-hydroxy-3-methyl" portion of the molecule name indicates that carbon 3 has both a hydroxy group and a methyl group (which is carbon #6) attached. The "yl" ending indicates a functional group joined to another functional group. Thus pick one of the carboxylic acid groups and attach it in a thioester bond to coenzyme A. This reaction is joining two molecules to form a larger molecule. The enzyme will then be either a *synthase* (no ATP used) or a *synthetase* (ATP used). This reaction does <u>not</u> use ATP, so the enzyme is a *synthase*. Synthases (and synthetases) are named for the <u>product</u>. Therefore the enzyme is called **HMG-CoA synthase**.

In reaction #3, a molecule of acetyl CoA is clipped off, which seems a bit wasteful because reaction #2 just added a third acetyl CoA. However, the formation of HMG-CoA is what drives the thiolase reaction (reaction #1) to run in "reverse" to make the acetoacetyl CoA. In reaction #3, the acetyl CoA molecule is clipped off by **HMG-CoA lyase** to end up with the 4-carbon product acetoacetate. Note that it looks like acetoacetyl CoA, without the "CoA" attached. Note the carbon numbering on acetoacetate. The methyl group (carbon #4) of acetoacetate was the methyl group (carbon #6) of HMG-CoA. The molecular name "acetoacetate" indicates its structure: two acetyl groups attached together. **Acetoacetate** is the first ketone body formed.

Figure 4.7: Pathway of ketone body synthesis (3 to 4 steps)

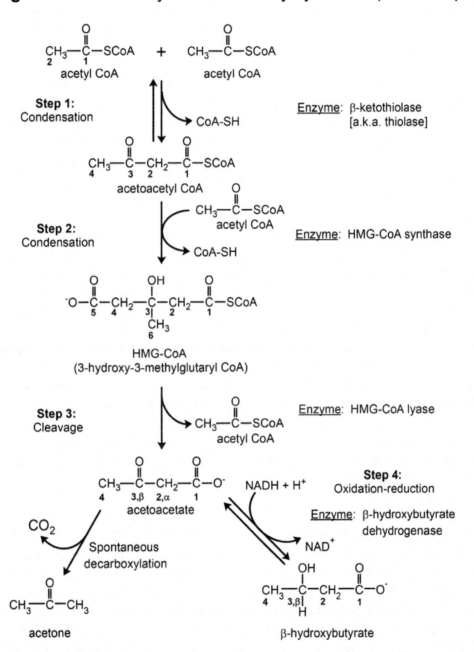

Consider the structure of acetoacetate. It is a β-ketoacid, which means the carboxylic acid group can spontaneously decarboxylate to form CO_2. Again, spontaneously does not mean instantaneously. As molecules of acetoacetate travel through the bloodstream, a proportion of them will spontaneously decarboxylate to form **acetone**, another ketone body. The structure of acetone was initially introduced in chapter 1 as part of the oxidation states flow chart (**Figure 1.7**). Tissues cannot use acetone as a fuel source because it cannot be converted back to two molecules of acetyl CoA. Thus, acetone is excreted from the body, either by breathing it off from the lungs or in the urine.

To allow more of the ketone bodies to be used as a fuel source rather than excreted, this pathway includes a fourth reaction that reduces the β-keto group of acetoacetate to a secondary alcohol, forming β-hydroxybutyrate. This ketone body, **β-hydroxybutyrate**, is four carbons as indicate by the prefix "but" (means "four" in organic chemistry nomenclature). The "-ate" ending indicates the deprotonated carboxylic acid group on an end carbon (carbon #1), with a hydroxy on the β-carbon (carbon #3). This ketone body is the only ketone body that does not have a keto group.

The formation of β-hydroxybutyrate is a reduction reaction, so there must be a simultaneous oxidation reaction. Since the reduction from a ketone to an alcohol is going "up" the oxidation states flow chart (**Figure 1.7**), one would expect NADPH + H$^+$ to be reduced to NADP$^+$. This reaction is occurring in the mitochondrial matrix, though. NADPH is the form of reducing power used for synthetic reactions, which usually occur in the cytosol, and NADPH is not capable of giving its electrons to the ETC. NADH is the more available form of reducing power in the matrix, and therefore this reaction uses NADH +H$^+$ and oxidizes it to NAD$^+$ in this reaction. Enzymes that catalyze oxidation-reduction reactions using NAD$^+$ or FAD are called *dehydrogenases*. Dehydrogenases are named for the <u>more reduced</u> molecule, β-hydroxybutyrate. The enzyme that catalyzes reaction #4 is called **β-hydroxybutyrate dehydrogenase**. This reaction is reversible, and the β-hydroxybutyrate dehydrogenase enzyme of the tissues that take up ketone bodies do the reverse reaction to oxidize β-hydroxybutyrate back to acetoacetate, and simultaneously reduce NAD$^+$ to NADH + H$^+$.

The amount of acetoacetate that is reduced to β-hydroxybutyrate by the liver is dependent upon the ratio of NADH/NAD$^+$ in the matrix. The more NADH that is available the more acetoacetate molecules can be reduced to β-hydroxybutyrate. This reduced form, β-hydroxybutyrate, is the ketone body that is preferred for circulation in the blood because it cannot spontaneously decarboxylate like acetoacetate can. Thus more ketone bodies are available for use by the tissues. Of the three ketone bodies, β-hydroxybutyrate does not have a keto group. Certain clinical tests that rely on a reaction with a keto group, i.e. reaction with sodium nitroprusside, will only detect acetoacetate and acetone. While the test will not detect the β-hydroxybutyrate, presumably the more prevalent ketone body in circulation in the blood, one can infer the relative amounts of ketone bodies based on the amounts of acetoacetate and acetone detected.

CONDITIONS UNDER WHICH KETONE BODIES ARE PRODUCED BY THE LIVER

A metabolic priority of the liver is to provide water-soluble fuel sources, in the form of glucose and ketone bodies, as readily available fuel sources (or "fast food") for tissues to use. Glucose is preferred by the brain, and a necessity for mature red blood cells. Under conditions where the liver is maintaining blood glucose by *de novo* synthesis through gluconeogenesis, ketone body synthesis is also up-regulated. The brain can use ketone bodies as a fuel source, though usually after about 48 hours of starvation. Under starvation conditions, other tissues preferentially begin to utilize ketone bodies to reserve the available glucose for the brain and red blood cells.

The entry of acetyl CoA into the TCA cycle depends on the presence of oxaloacetate. Recall that oxaloacetate concentrations are kept low in the cell. Oxaloacetate is used almost as quickly as it is made. Oxaloacetate can be formed directly from pyruvate by pyruvate carboxylase (the first enzyme of gluconeogenesis) or from malate by malate dehydrogenase (the last step of the TCA cycle). When oxaloacetate is made it is used— either by citrate synthase of the TCA cycle, or reduced by malate dehydrogenase during gluconeogenesis. In the case of ketone body synthesis, the "low" concentrations of oxaloacetate means that oxaloacetate is not available for citrate synthase to use to run the TCA cycle. Under conditions when the cell is doing gluconeogenesis, oxaloacetate is formed from pyruvate carboxylase and citrate synthase is inhibited. The oxaloacetate is being reduced to malate, which is then transported to the cytosol for gluconeogenesis to continue in the cytosol. Under these condition pyruvate carboxylase is active and the PDH complex is turned off. These are two enzymes in the same compartment that use the same substrate, pyruvate. The PDH complex and pyruvate carboxylase are regulated by high mitochondrial concentrations of acetyl CoA. The acetyl CoA used for ketone body synthesis comes from β-oxidation of fatty acids. As discussed, the catabolism of fatty acids yields much more acetyl CoA molecules than the catabolism of glucose.

Under what conditions (i.e. when?), then, would oxaloacetate concentrations be low in the matrix (i.e. unavailable for use by the TCA cycle)? A low carbohydrate diet forces the liver to make glucose via gluconeogenesis to maintain blood glucose for other tissues, as would starvation conditions when a person is not eating anything. Uncontrolled diabetic conditions also result in the liver production of glucose and ketone bodies. There may be plenty of glucose in the blood, but without insulin the liver cannot detect the blood glucose levels. Therefore the liver continues to secrete glucose and ketone bodies into the blood. Under these three conditions, gluconeogenesis is predominating in the liver to form glucose because it is a metabolic priority.

Under these conditions, there is no oxaloacetate available in the matrix to run the TCA cycle. As gluconeogenesis is up-regulated in the liver, the catabolism of triacylglycerols from adipose cells is activated to provide fatty acids to the liver (via circulation in the blood attached to albumin). The fatty acids are transported into the mitochondrial matrix by the carnitine shuttle where they are catabolized to acetyl CoA by β-oxidation. As the oxaloacetate formed is now an intermediate of gluconeogenesis and not available for the citrate synthase reaction of the TCA cycle, the acetyl CoA produced by β-oxidation is used for ketone body synthesis.

In the liver, the excess acetyl CoA formed by β-oxidation also simultaneously regulates two enzymes in the mitochondrial matrix that both use pyruvate as a substrate. A high concentration of acetyl CoA in the matrix inhibits the pyruvate dehydrogenase (PDH) complex, the bridging step between glycolysis and the TCA cycle. High concentrations of acetyl CoA in the matrix simultaneously activates pyruvate carboxylase, the first enzyme of gluconeogenesis. This simultaneous regulation of two enzymes that use the same substrate directs the use of pyruvate under conditions of excess acetyl CoA towards production of glucose via gluconeogenesis. The excess acetyl CoA from β-oxidation is then used for ketone body synthesis. Thus, the liver does gluconeogenesis and ketone body synthesis to provide the necessary water-soluble fuel sources to the blood for use by other tissues.

FATES OF KETONE BODIES

The three ketone bodies are acetoacetate, β-hydroxybutyrate, and acetone. They are water-soluble, which means they do not need a transporter for circulation in the blood. Both acetoacetate and β-hydroxybutyrate are four carbons. The tissues that take them up can convert them back to two molecules of acetyl CoA. The tissues that take up ketone bodies can convert them to acetyl CoA, which they can use for whatever they want (i.e. TCA cycle, fatty acid synthesis, cholesterol synthesis)—but not ketone body synthesis, which can only be done in the liver. Acetone, on the other hand, is only three carbons. Acetone is excreted. Acetone can be expired through the lungs, as it is volatile, and it can be excreted in the urine as well. Acetone is the molecule that produces the "fruity breath" smell from a person who is experiencing ketoacidosis due to uncontrolled diabetes. If ketone bodies are produced excessively, then all three ketone bodies can be excreted in the urine.

Tissues, such as skeletal muscle tissue, that take up acetoacetate and β-hydroxybutyrate convert them back to two molecules of acetyl CoA, as briefly described. The ketone body β-hydroxybutyrate is first oxidized back to acetoacetate by *β-hydroxybutyrate dehydrogenase*, with simultaneous reduction of NAD^+ to $NADH + H^+$ (i.e. the reverse reaction of Step 4 in **Figure 4.7**). Molecules of acetoacetate are then attached to coenzyme A to form acetoacetyl CoA. The donor of coenzyme A is succinyl CoA, an intermediate of the TCA cycle. The removal of coenzyme A from succinyl CoA forms succinate, another intermediate of the TCA cycle. The enzyme that carries out this reaction is *β-ketoacyl CoA transferase*. This is the enzyme that liver cells lack, which prevents the liver from using ketone bodies as a fuel source. Now the molecules of acetoacetyl CoA can be cleaved to form two molecules of acetyl CoA by *β-ketothiolase*, also known as *acetoacetyl CoA thiolase* in this pathway. This is the same enzyme, though, that carries out this reaction during step 4 of the four repeated steps of β-oxidation of fatty acids.

When ketone body synthesis exceeds the rate at which they are used by the tissues, this excess ketone body production is called *ketosis*. The levels of ketone bodies begin to rise in the blood, referred to as *ketonemia*, and ultimately are excreted in excess in the urine, referred to as *ketonuria*. Excess ketone body production leads to what is called *ketoacidosis*. These molecules have carboxylic acids that deprotonate and contribute protons to the blood. Increasing proton concentration causes the blood pH to drop and become more acidic. Ketoacidosis is usually seen in uncontrolled type I diabetics, where ketone bodies are produced in excess, and are not adequately taken up by tissues in relation to their production.

CHAPTER 5: FATTY ACID SYNTHESIS

Objectives:

1. Define the process of fatty acid synthesis.
2. Explain the purpose of the pathway of fatty acid synthesis, and why linoleic and linolenic acids are essential fatty acids.
   a. Calculate how many cycles of the four repeated steps of fatty acid synthesis are necessary to generate the major product—palmitate ($C_{16:0}$ fatty acid).
   b. Explain, in general terms, how longer-chain fatty acids (C_{18} and higher) are synthesized and how double bonds are introduced into the acyl chain.
   c. Explain why linoleic and linolenic acids are dietary requirements.
3. Identify where fatty acid synthesis takes place in the cell.
   a. Explain how acetyl CoA, which is produced in the mitochondrial matrix, is shuttled out to the cytosol, and why a special export mechanism is required.
4. Explain how fatty acid synthesis is carried out in the cell.
   a. Identify the "committed step" of fatty acid synthesis, the enzyme that catalyzes this step and its regulatory effectors.
   b. Describe the four "main" repeated steps of fatty acid synthesis, and identify the enzymes and cofactor(s) involved.
   c. Explain the advantages of having all the enzymes involved in fatty acid synthesis (except acetyl CoA carboxylase) bound together in one large complex, and the role the phosphopantetheine group plays in the synthesis process.
5. Explain when fatty acid synthesis takes place.
   a. Identify the regulatory enzymes of fatty acid synthesis, what regulates them, and how hormones regulate fatty acid synthesis.
6. Compare and contrast the overall similarities and differences of the reciprocal pathways of fatty oxidation and fatty acid synthesis
   a. Compare and contrast the overall similarities and differences of the reciprocal pathways of fatty oxidation and fatty acid synthesis—including substrates, products, cofactors, enzymes and regulation of the pathways.

FATTY ACID SYNTHESIS

The name of this pathway tells you its definition (what?). Fatty acid synthesis is the synthesis of fatty acids from acetyl CoA. The typical fatty acid synthesized by the fatty acid synthase complex is palmitic acid (or palmitate, as the deprotonated form), a 16-carbon saturate fatty acid. Note that just like gluconeogenesis is not an exact reversal of glycolysis, neither is fatty acid synthesis an exact reversal of β-oxidation.

The fatty acids synthesized can be used for a variety of complex lipid syntheses (why?). For instance, fatty acids are components of membrane lipids, triacylglycerols, and lipoproteins. Fatty acids, though, are not going to be synthesized to send into the mitochondria for immediate breakdown by β-oxidation because that would be a futile cycle. A liver cell is not going to synthesize a fatty acid and then use it for ketone body synthesis because β-oxidation precedes ketone body synthesis. So fatty acid synthesis and β-oxidation are reciprocal pathways that cannot occur in the same cell at the same time. There are distinct regulators that prevent these two pathways from being active at the same time in the same cell.

Figure 5.1: The net reaction of palmitate (C_{16}) synthesis and malonyl CoA synthesis

Palmitate synthesis

1 acetyl CoA + 7 malonyl CoA +
14 NADPH + 20 H^+ $\longrightarrow$ 1 palmitate + 7 CO_2 + 8 CoA +
14 $NADP^+$ + 6 H_2O

Malonyl CoA synthesis

7 acetyl CoA + 7 CO_2 + 7 ATP $\longrightarrow$ 7 malonyl CoA + 7 ADP + 7 P_i + 14 H^+

Fatty acid synthesis occurs in the cytosol of cells (where?). The net reaction for fatty acid synthesis of palmitate is shown in **Figure 5.1**. Fatty acid synthesis uses only one actual molecule of acetyl CoA and then 7 malonyl CoA to synthesize a molecule of palmitate, which is a 16-carbon saturated fatty acid. As one should expect in a synthetic pathway, a lot of reducing power in the form of NADPH is required. However, there is not ATP shown in this net reaction. Synthetic pathways should require an input of energy to make larger molecules from small starting units. The actual enzyme complex that attaches the 2-carbon units together and does the necessary reductions and dehydration reaction does not require ATP, as one could deduce from the name of the enzyme complex—the fatty acid *synthase* complex. Synthases are enzymes that do not require energy. There is one enzyme involved in fatty acid synthesis, though, that is <u>not</u> part of the complex. Acetyl CoA carboxylase synthesizes malonyl CoA by carboxylation of acetyl CoA and requires ATP. The net reaction for malonyl CoA synthesis is also shown in **Figure 5.1**. Only one acetyl CoA molecule is needed per fatty acid synthesized, the remaining 2-carbon units are attached using malonyl CoA. The synthesis of malonyl CoA must be done first to create a pool of malonyl CoA molecules for use by the fatty acid synthase complex, which is the energy requiring step.

This pathway is a little more complicated than the catabolism of fatty acids (β-oxidation). One can think about this pathway as similar to an assembly line for car manufacturing. A car is built on an assembly line where parts of the car are added at each step before the entire car is "released" from the assembly line. The fatty acid synthase complex works the same way. All of the intermediates are added and reduced to the level of an alkane by the enzymes of the fatty acid synthase complex before the complete molecule of palmitate is released from the complex.

Figure 5.2: Overview of fatty acid synthesis

FIRST: Transport acetyl CoA from the mitochondrial matrix to the cytosol by way of citrate (using malate/citrate/pyruvate shuttle).
SECOND: Acetyl CoA is carboxylated to form malonyl CoA by the enzyme *acetyl CoA carboxylase*.
THIRD: Chain growth by head-to-tail condensation and reduction to an alkane by the enzymes of the fatty acid synthase complex.

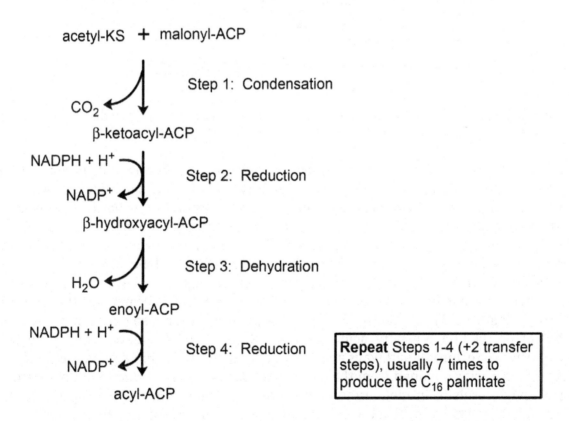

The overview of the pathway of fatty acid synthesis is shown in **Figure 5.2**. For learning the process (how?) of fatty acid synthesis, one needs to know how molecules of acetyl CoA, which are generated in the mitochondrial matrix, are transported into the cytosol. A pool of malonyl CoA will then be produced from the acetyl CoA. For fatty acid synthesis there are 6 repeated steps that are carried out in the production of palmitate. Two of the steps are "transfer steps" to correctly position the growing fatty acid and a new molecule of malonyl CoA for continued lengthening of the carbon chain. There are four repeated steps that one should compare and contrast to the four repeated steps of β-oxidation of fatty acids, which will be referred to subsequently as the four "key" repeated steps. These four keys steps of focus for this pathway, shown in the overview diagram for this pathway (**Figure 5.2**), correspond to moving "up" the oxidation states flow chart (**Figure 1.7**) to go from a more oxidized state of carbon to a more reduced state of carbon. In fact, exercise #5 at the end of the chapter 1 (the oxidation states chapter) required one to put in order the correct sequence of molecules for the first three reactions (of the 4 key repeated steps) of fatty acid synthesis based on their structures, and name the enzymes for these reactions.

Figure 5.3: Sources and uses of acetyl CoA.

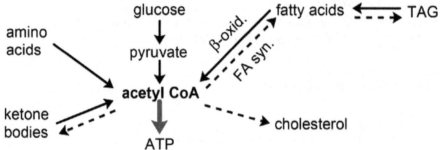

[Note: Acetyl CoA is used for ATP production via the TCA cycle and the reducing power that is sent to the electron transport chain.]

Figure 5.3 indicates the sources and uses of acetyl CoA. Excess nutrients in the diet (i.e. sugars and amino acids) can be converted to fatty acids for storage on triacylglycerols. Glycolysis and the PDH complex will yield a source of acetyl CoA that can be used for fatty acid synthesis. Tissues that take up ketone bodies could also use the acetyl CoA formed from them for fatty acid synthesis. The catabolism of some amino acids from protein breakdown may also yield acetyl CoA, which could be used for fatty acid synthesis by the cell. Acetyl CoA can be used to make cholesterol, as well, but cholesterol cannot be catabolized back to acetyl CoA (as indicated by the one-way arrow in **Figure 5.3**). Catabolism of fatty acids by β-oxidation also does not provide the pool of acetyl CoA for fatty acid synthesis. Recall that β-oxidation and fatty acid synthesis are reciprocal pathways and will not be "on" at the same time in the same cell. Excess fatty acids obtained from the diet can be used for the production of body stores of triacylglycerols or in membrane lipid synthesis. If one thinks of the function of the liver, it is trying to store all of the excess nutrients obtained from the diet. The liver only stores a certain amount of glycogen, as a readily accessible source of glucose. For an adult, the liver stores about a 24-hour supply of glucose in the form of glycogen. The remaining excess nutrients are stored as triacylglycerols, 3 fatty acids attached to a glycerol backbone.

Triacylglycerols (TAGs or fat) are the most efficient storage form of fuel, as discussed previously, and are not rapidly mobilized. TAGs can be stored for 150 days or longer. Glycogen is storage form of glucose to supply a ready source of glucose, particularly for catabolism to produce ATP. As the liver is the primary organ responsible for maintaining blood glucose, its glycogen stores are the only glycogen stores that can release glucose for use by all other tissues. However, an adult liver can only store about a 24-hour supply of glucose. Proteins in the body are constantly turned over (particular enzymes), but proteins are not an "energy source" that is regularly used by cells. There is no protein whose sole function is to serve as an "energy store" for the cell like glycogen and triacylglycerols. When any protein is broken down, while it does can yield ATP by further catabolizing the amino acid components, the actual function of that protein is "lost," whether it was a structural function (i.e. muscle), enzymatic, or transporter as examples. Some of the longer-functioning proteins are turned over in a maximum of about 10 days.

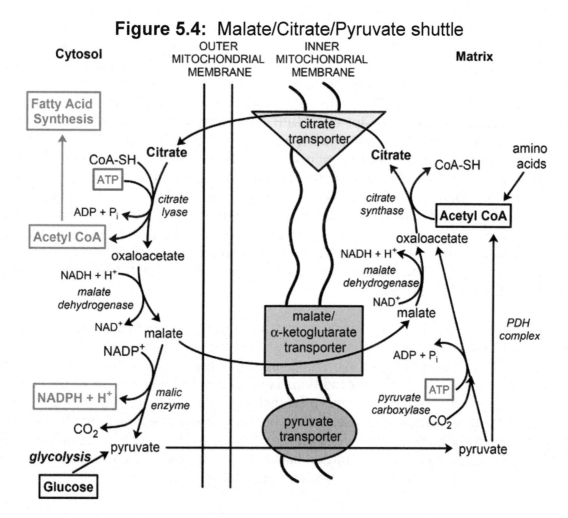

Figure 5.4: Malate/Citrate/Pyruvate shuttle

For the pathway of fatty acid synthesis, there is a transport issue that must first be discussed. The acetyl CoA produced for this pathway (i.e. from the PDH complex, amino acid catabolism, or the use of ketone bodies) is all produced in the mitochondrial matrix. Fatty acid synthesis takes place in the cytosol, so the acetyl CoA must be transported from the matrix to the cytosol. **Figure 5.4** shows the malate/citrate/pyruvate shuttle that is used to transport acetyl CoA from the matrix to the cytosol. In **Figure 5.4**, start with the acetyl CoA in the <u>matrix</u>, which comes from glucose (via glycolysis and the PDH complex) or amino acid catabolism. Under conditions where the cell needs to synthesize fatty acids, citrate synthase carries out the first reaction of the TCA cycle to form citrate from the condensation of acetyl CoA to oxaloacetate. Now, though, the citrate does not continue through the TCA cycle. Instead, the citrate is transported across the inner mitochondrial membrane (through a specific transporter) to ultimately end up in the cytosol. Citrate is, thus, the carrier of the acetyl CoA units to the cytosol. Once the citrate is in the cytosol, an enzyme called **citrate lyase** cleaves (i.e. "lyses") citrate to re-form acetyl CoA and oxaloacetate. Now a pool of acetyl CoA is available to be used for fatty acid synthesis or cholesterol synthesis, as both pathways take place in the cytosol of a cell.

As the TCA cycle is not running in the matrix under these conditions, the oxaloacetate formed in the cytosol needs to be transported back into the matrix. However, as previously discussed, oxaloacetate does not have a transporter in the inner mitochondrial membrane. Malate is allowed to cross, so the oxaloacetate can be reduced to malate by cytosolic malate dehydrogenase. Malate is then transported back to the matrix to be re-oxidized to oxaloacetate by mitochondrial malate dehydrogenase. Fatty acid synthesis requires a lot of NADPH, the form of reducing power needed to donate electrons for the reduction of molecules in synthetic processes. The majority of NADPH is produced by the pentose phosphate pathway. However, additional NADPH can be formed from another enzymatic reaction in this shuttle. A cytosolic enzyme called **malic enzyme** (which does not follow any of the naming rules, including the "-ase" ending used for enzymes) produces pyruvate from the decarboxylation and oxidation of malate. The purpose of this step produces additional molecules of NADPH needed for fatty acid synthesis. The ratio of the amount of malate versus pyruvate transported back to the matrix will depend on the ratio of NADPH/NADP$^+$ in the cytosol needed for fatty acid synthesis.

The pyruvate produced by malic enzymes can also be transported back into the matrix where it can be used to form more acetyl CoA (via the PDH complex) or oxaloacetate (via pyruvate carboxylase). The matrix having both the PDH complex and pyruvate carboxylase "active" under these conditions is a "complicating factor" to consider. One would not generally expect two enzymes that use the same substrate in the same cellular compartment, as in this case, to both be "on" at the same time. What happens to the pyruvate in the matrix will depend on the need for oxaloacetate based on the ratio of malate versus pyruvate being shuttled back into the matrix, as well as the amount of acetyl CoA that needs to be sent to cytosol for fatty acid synthesis.

The cell now has a pool of acetyl CoA in the cytosol. The first reaction of fatty acid synthesis, shown in **Figure 5.5**, is <u>not</u> part of the fatty acid synthase complex. This enzymatic reaction must create a pool of malonyl CoA molecules for use by the complex, first. The reaction is the carboxylation of acetyl CoA to form malonyl CoA, which requires energy in the form of ATP. The enzyme is a *carboxylase* and is named for the molecule accepting the molecule of CO_2, acetyl CoA. Therefore, the enzyme that catalyzes this reaction is called ***acetyl CoA carboxylase***.

Figure 5.5: Formation of malonyl CoA, the committed step in FA synthesis

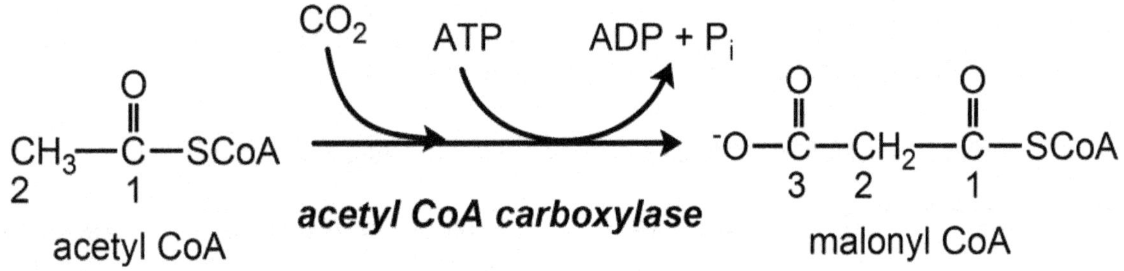

Carboxylase enzymes require the coenzyme, biotin. **Figure 5.6** shows the two steps of the carboxylase enzyme reaction using biotin as the coenzyme. Acetyl CoA carboxylase first picks up the CO_2 group (from bicarbonate, HCO_3^-) and attaches it to its biotin coenzyme. The carboxylic acid group is then transferred to the methyl carbon (carbon #2) of acetyl CoA to form malonyl CoA. Malonyl CoA is now three carbons containing a carboxylic acid group at each end. The carboxylic acid carbon that is designated carbon #1 of malonyl CoA, though, is the one that is joined to coenzyme A via a thioester bond (as shown in **Figure 5.5**).

Figure 5.6: The two steps of the acetyl CoA carboxylase reaction involving biotin

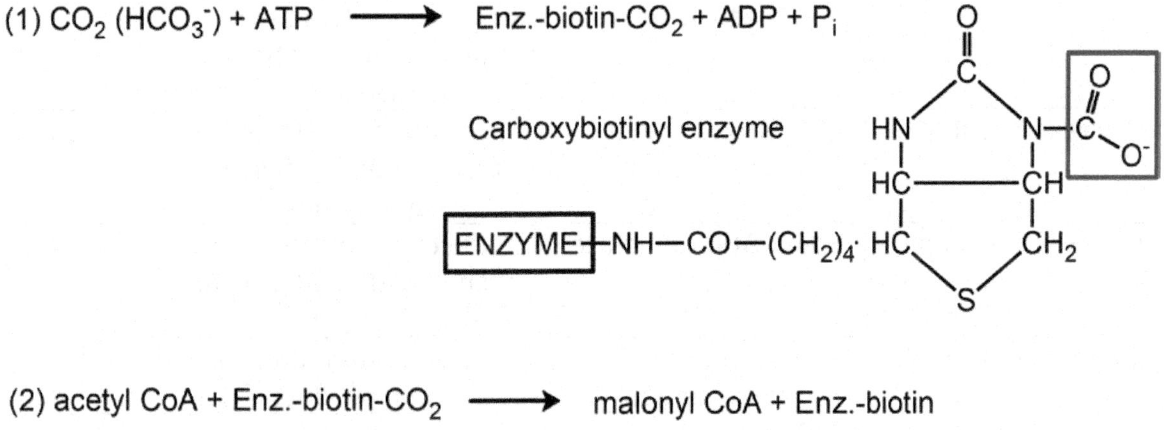

(1) CO_2 (HCO_3^-) + ATP $\longrightarrow$ Enz.-biotin-CO_2 + ADP + P_i

Carboxybiotinyl enzyme

(2) acetyl CoA + Enz.-biotin-CO_2 $\longrightarrow$ malonyl CoA + Enz.-biotin

The acetyl CoA carboxylase reaction is irreversible and the committed step of fatty acid synthesis. Thus, this is the key regulated step of the pathway. The removal of the carboxylic acid group (carbon #3) is what will drive the condensation reaction, the first reaction of the four key repeated steps of fatty acid synthesis.

The fatty acid synthase (FAS) complex is very large. In humans (and other vertebrates), the fatty acid synthase complex is a dimer of two identical subunits that lie head-to-tail relative to one another. Each subunit of the dimer is composed of a single large polypeptide containing all seven enzymes (i.e. 2 transfer step enzymes, the 4 enzymes for the 4 "key" repeated catalytic steps, as well as the enzyme that clips off the final product). See **Table 5.1** for a list of all 7 enzymes and the reactions they carry out. Note that the name of the complex is a *synthase*, which are enzymes that do not use energy in the form of ATP. The synthase is named for the <u>product</u> of the complex—a fatty acid. Thus the complex is called the ***fatty acid synthase complex***.

Table 5.1: The enzymatic components of the fatty acid synthase complex

Step	Component	Reaction/Function	Repeated Step
Transfer step 1	Acetyl CoA-ACP transacylase	Transfers first acetyl CoA or growing acyl chains to the cysteine of the β-ketoacyl-ACP synthase	Yes
Transfer step 2	Malonyl CoA-ACP transacylase	Transfers malonyl units onto the sulfhydryl group of the ACP	Yes
Key reaction step 3	β-ketoacyl-ACP synthase (a.k.a. the condensing enzyme)	Condenses the acetyl unit or growing acyl chain onto carbon 2 of the malonyl units on the ACP, with loss of CO_2	Yes
Key reaction step 4	β-ketoacyl-ACP reductase	Reduces the keto group on the β-carbon to a hydroxy group, with oxidation of NADPH	Yes
Key reaction step 5	β-hydroxyacyl-ACP dehydratase	Dehydrates to form a *trans*-alkene between carbons 2 and 3.	Yes
Key reaction step 6	Enoyl-ACP reductase	Reduces the alkene to an alkane, with oxidation of NADPH.	Yes
Final reaction step 7	palmitoyl thioesterase	Clips off palmitate, the final product	No

The fatty acid synthase complex also has an **acyl carrier protein**, abbreviated ACP. The acyl carrier protein is derived from pantothenic acid (like coenzyme A). The acyl carrier protein has a free sulfhydryl group (-SH) at its terminus. Acyl groups are attached to the ACP via a thioester bond, in the same manner fatty acids are attached to coenzyme A molecules. The acyl carrier protein serves as a "long arm" that can reach all of the enzyme active sites of the complex. The function of the ACP, then, is to carry the acyl intermediates around to each enzyme of the complex for the subsequent rounds of the four key repeated steps of fatty acid synthesis.

There are two transfer steps that are repeated (see **Table 5.1**). These two transfer steps are to place the initial acetyl CoA for the first round of repeated steps (or the growing acyl chain in the following rounds) onto a cysteine group of the β-ketoacyl-ACP synthase (after the 4th step of the four key repeated steps), such that the malonyl unit is always transferred onto the sulfhydryl group of the ACP. The condensation of the growing acyl chain onto the new malonyl unit allows the new chain to end up on the ACP for the remaining 3 steps, as the ACP can carry it to the other enzyme active sites. The four key repeated steps that coincide with going "up" the oxidation states flow chart (**Figure 1.7**) are the focus, and are shown in **Figure 5.7**.

Figure 5.7 shows the 4 key repeated steps of fatty acid synthesis. These are the four steps one should be able to compare and contrast with the pathway of β-oxidation. The reactions of the fatty acid synthase complex begin with the transfer steps, which are not shown in **Figure 5.7**. *Acetyl CoA-ACP transacylase* transfers the 2-carbon unit from a molecule of acetyl CoA to the –SH group of a cysteine residue of the β-ketoacyl-ACP synthase, abbreviated KS. The acetyl unit is shown attached to "KS" as a starting material of step 1 in **Figure 5.7**. The 3-carbon unit from a molecule of malonyl CoA is then transferred to the –SH group of the acyl carrier protein (ACP) by the enzyme *malonyl CoA-ACP transacylase*. In **Figure 5.7**, the malonyl unit is shown attached to the ACP as the other starting material of step 1.

In the pathway of β-oxidation, the four repeated steps were oxidation to an alkene, hydration to a secondary alcohol, oxidation to a keto group, then cleave off an acetyl CoA. In fatty acid synthesis, two 2-carbon units need to be connected together, first, to create a 4-carbon molecule. The first key reaction, as shown in **Figure 5.7**, is a condensation reaction—the attachment of the two 2-carbon units together. In this reaction, the decarboxylation of the malonyl unit (the carbon #3 carboxylic acid group) drives the condensation of the acetyl unit **onto** carbon #2 of the malonyl unit. (In subsequent rounds, it will be the growing acyl chain that condenses onto carbon #2 of the new malonyl unit.) The product of this first condensation reaction is a 4-carbon intermediate attached to the acyl carrier protein, called β-ketoacyl ACP.

This reaction involves attaching two molecules together to make a larger molecule. Recall that enzymes that catalyze synthesis reactions are called synthases or synthetases, depending on whether or not ATP is used, and are named for the product of the reaction. As this reaction does not require ATP, the enzyme is called a *synthase*, and the product is β-ketoacyl ACP. Therefore, the enzyme for reaction #1 is called *β-ketoacyl-ACP synthase*. This "ACP" as part of the enzyme names of the fatty acid synthase complex should serve as one way to easily distinguish the names of enzymes of the four repeated steps of fatty acid synthesis versus β-oxidation. The β-ketoacyl-ACP synthase enzyme is often referred to as the "*condensing enzyme*."

Figure 5.7: The four "key" repeated steps of the fatty acid synthase complex.

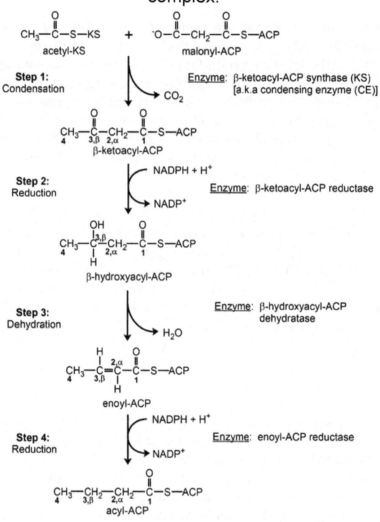

REPEAT Steps 1-4 (+2 transfer steps), usually 7 times producing palmitate ($C_{16:0}$).

[Note: There are actually 6 repeated steps for each 2 carbon addition. The other 2 steps are "transfer" steps: First—to move the growing acyl chain back to the sulfhydryl group of the condensing enzyme; Second—to bring on the next malonyl group to the acyl carrier protein (ACP). **Also note** that all subsequent 2 carbon additions come from **malonyl CoA**. The only acetyl CoA used is in the first round.]

This 4-carbon product of reaction #1 looks like a β-ketoacyl CoA intermediate of β-oxidation (i.e. the product of reaction #3 in β-oxidation), only now the 4-carbon unit is attached to the acyl carrier protein instead of coenzyme A. Recall the purpose of this pathway is to make a 16-carbon saturated fatty acid. Fatty acids have only one carboxylic acid group at carbon #1. The remaining carbons are all at the level of an alkane for a saturated fatty acid. In looking at the structure of the product, β-ketoacyl ACP, the keto group on carbon #3 (the β-carbon) needs to be reduced back to the level of an alkane. According to the oxidation states flow chart (**Figure 1.7**), the reaction sequence needed to accomplish this is to reduce the keto group to a secondary alcohol, dehydrate to form an alkene, then reduce the alkene to an alkane. The next three enzymes of the fatty acid synthase complex carry out these exact three reactions.

The second key reaction, shown in **Figure 5.7**, is the reduction of the β-keto group (carbon #3) on the β-ketoacyl ACP to a secondary alcohol, forming β-hydroxyacyl ACP. The reduction reaction requires a simultaneous oxidation reaction. When going "up" the oxidation states flow chart, NADPH + H+ is the form of reducing power used, and it will be oxidized to NADP+. Enzymes that catalyze oxidation-reduction reactions using NADP+ or NADPH, regardless of which direction the reaction is going, are called *reductases*. Reductases are named for the more oxidized molecule because that is what is being reduced. In this reaction, the β-ketoacyl ACP molecule is more oxidized, so the enzyme is called ***β-ketoacyl-ACP reductase***.

In step #3 (**Figure 5.7**), a molecule of water is removed (i.e. dehydration) from the β-hydroxyacyl ACP to form an alkene between carbons #2 and #3 in the product, enoyl ACP. This is also a *trans* double bond, like in β-oxidation, and will be removed in the following step. The enzyme that catalyzes this dehydration reaction is called a *dehydratase*, and it is named for the molecule that is losing the water—β-hydroxyacyl ACP. The enzyme is called ***β-hydroxyacyl-ACP dehydratase***.

Step #4 (**Figure 5.7**) now reduces the alkene (enoyl ACP) to an alkane, forming an acyl ACP. For this reduction the form of reducing power is still NADPH + H+, which will get oxidized to NADP+. An enzyme that catalyzes an oxidation-reduction reaction using NADPH is called a *reductase*. A reductase is named for the more oxidized molecule, which is enoyl ACP for this reaction. This enzyme is called ***enoyl-ACP reductase.*** This product is now a 4-carbon fatty acid attached to the acyl carrier protein of the complex.

Before another 2-carbon unit can be added, the ***acetyl CoA-ACP transacylase*** transfers this 4-carbon acyl unit to the –SH group on the cysteine residue of the β-ketoacyl ACP synthase enzyme. Then the ***malonyl CoA-ACP transacylase*** brings on the 3-carbon unit from a new malonyl CoA molecule and attaches it to the -SH group of the acyl carrier protein (ACP). Note that for all subsequent rounds of fatty acid synthesis, malonyl CoA is the donor of the 2-carbon units. The only actual molecule of acetyl CoA used is in the first round. The β-ketoacyl ACP synthase then condenses the 4-carbon acyl unit onto carbon #2 of the new malonyl unit, with the loss of CO_2. Now a 6-carbon unit has been formed that has a beta-keto group that needs to be reduced back to an alkane by reduction, dehydration, and reduction. In subsequent rounds of fatty acid synthesis, the acetyl CoA-ACP transacylase will move the growing acyl chain (after step 4) from the ACP to the cysteine residue of the β-ketoacyl-ACP synthase. This will allow the new malonyl unit to always be transferred to the ACP by malonyl CoA-ACP transacylase. Note that the names of these transfer enzymes indicate the reactions they carry out.

It requires 7 cycles of these 4 repeated steps (6-repeated steps when including the two transfer steps) to produce the typical product, palmitate, a 16-carbon saturated fatty acid. When the 16-carbon fatty acid has been formed, the enzyme **palmitoyl thioesterase** cleaves the thioester bond that attaches the acyl group to the ACP, forming palmitate. Palmitate will then be attached to coenzyme A, forming palmitoyl CoA, by the enzyme fatty acyl CoA synthetase (**Figure 4.3**). Fatty acids must always be attached to a carrier, as previously discussed.

Palmitate is not the only fatty acid in the body, though it is the major product of the fatty acid synthase complex. Further processing of fatty acids occurs in the endoplasmic reticulum. Longer fatty acids can be produced (i.e. 18-carbons, 20-carbons, etc.) by elongating palmitate (or other fatty acids) using molecules of malonyl CoA as the 2-carbon donor, similar to the fatty acid synthase complex. Malonyl CoA is used to sequentially add 2-carbons to the **carboxyl end** of both saturated and unsaturated fatty acids.

Desaturation reactions can occur to introduce one or more **_cis_** double bonds (i.e. alkenes) to form unsaturated fatty acids. Recall that cis double bonds produce a bend or "kink" in the acyl chain of a fatty acid, preventing tight packing of fatty acids—especially in the membranes. The reactions to make double bonds are carried out by several enzymes (termed mixed-function oxidases) including a reductase and a desaturase. One or more _cis_-double bonds can be introduced at various positions along the acyl chain.

Humans, however, cannot introduce double bonds past carbon #9 of a fatty acid. Since palmitate is the primary product of the fatty acid synthase complex and humans do not have enzymes capable of introducing double bonds past carbon #9, linoleic (ω-6) and linolenic (ω-3) fatty acids are essential fatty acids. Linoleic acid ($C_{18:2}^{\Delta 9,12}$) is an 18-carbon fatty acid with double bonds at carbon #9 and #12 (i.e. between carbons 9 and 10; and between carbons 12 and 13). Linolenic acid ($C_{18:3}^{\Delta 9,12,15}$) is an 18-carbon fatty acid with 3 double bonds at carbons 9, 12, and 15. Humans must obtain these fatty acids in the diet. The omega-3 fatty acids, like linolenic acid, are typically found in fish oils. The omega-6 fatty acids, like linoleic acid, are usually found in seed oils (i.e. vegetable oils). By obtaining these two essential fatty acids in the diet, the cells can further modify these fatty acids to produce other important fatty acids. Arachidonate ($C_{20:4}^{\Delta 5,8,11,14}$) is a 20-carbon fatty acid with four double bonds synthesized from linoleic acid. Eicosapentaenoic acid (EPA), $C_{20:5}^{\Delta 5,8,11,14,17}$, is derived from linolenic acid. Both arachidonate and EPA are "stored" in membranes as part of various membrane phospholipids and help regulate membrane fluidity. The release of arachidonate or EPA leads to the production of different sets of eicosanoid hormones (i.e. prostaglandins, leukotrienes, and thromboxanes). The various eicosanoid hormones mediate numerous physiological processes such as smooth muscle contraction, regulation of blood flow, inflammation, fever, pain perception, and platelet aggregation.

REGULATION OF FATTY ACID SYNTHESIS

The regulation of the fatty acid synthesis pathway begins with the committed step, catalyzed by acetyl CoA carboxylase (the enzyme that is not part of the fatty acid synthase complex). It is regulated by hormones, such as insulin and glucagon. Insulin will activate the carboxylase, as expected. Insulin is an indicator of the fed state, allowing excess nutrients to be stored as triacylglycerols, for example. Glucagon inhibits the acetyl CoA carboxylase. Under these conditions, the liver (as a primary target tissue of glucagon) would be doing gluconeogenesis and ketone body synthesis to release water-soluble fuel sources into the blood. The acetyl CoA for ketone body synthesis comes from β-oxidation under these conditions. Fatty acid synthesis would be inhibited in a cell that is doing β-oxidation.

Citrate is an allosteric activator of acetyl CoA carboxylase. As citrate is the carrier of acetyl CoA units to the cytosol from the matrix, citrate is a cellular indicator that ATP and building blocks are abundant for fatty acid synthesis to occur. Palmitoyl CoA inhibits the acetyl CoA carboxylase. If palmitoyl CoA is abundant in the cytosol, it generally means that either fatty acids are being cut off of lipids (i.e. TAGs or phospholipids) or are being brought into the cell to serve as a fuel source. Under these conditions, these fatty acyl CoA molecules are being transported into the matrix for β-oxidation to occur, and thus fatty acid synthesis would be inhibited at the acetyl CoA carboxylase reaction. AMP also serves as an inhibitor of acetyl CoA carboxylase because high levels of AMP mean ATP levels are low. ATP is needed for synthesis of fatty acids.

Table 5.2: Reciprocal Regulation of FA oxidation and FA synthesis pathways

	Substrate	Regulated Enzyme	Regulators
β-oxidation	Palmitoyl CoA	Carnitine acyl transferase I (CAT I)	Malonyl CoA (−) Insulin (−) Glucagon (+)
FA synthesis	Malonyl CoA	acetyl CoA carboxylase	Palmitoyl CoA (−) Insulin (+) Glucagon (−)

Table 5.2 summarizes the reciprocal regulation of the two pathways of β-oxidation and fatty acid synthesis. Palmitoyl CoA, as previously mentioned, is an inhibitor fatty acid synthesis by inhibiting acetyl CoA carboxylase. Malonyl CoA, the main substrate for fatty acid synthesis, is an inhibitor of β-oxidation, specifically by inhibiting carnitine acyl transferase I (CAT I). Insulin, as a hormonal signal of the "fed" state, results in the dephosphorylation of key metabolic enzymes of target tissues, typically to active them.

Glucagon, as a hormonal indicator of low blood glucose, leads to the phosphorylation of key metabolic enzymes in its target tissues, typically to inactive them. Under insulin conditions, the cells can take up nutrients and do synthetic processes, like fatty acid synthesis, because fuel sources are readily abundant. For fatty acid synthesis, insulin dephosphorylates acetyl CoA carboxylase to activate it and activate fatty acid synthesis. The increase in concentration of malonyl CoA in the cytosol by acetyl CoA carboxylase inhibits CAT I, preventing fatty acids from entering the mitochondrial matris and as a result β-oxidation is inhibited.

When glucagon is the predominate hormone, the liver—a primary target tissue of glucagon, needs to release water-soluble fuel sources into the blood in the form of glucose and ketone bodies. Glucagon leads to the phosphorylation of acetyl CoA carboxylase, inhibiting it and fatty acid synthesis overall. The decrease in malonyl CoA in the cytosol relieves the inhibition of CAT I, allowing the influx of fatty acids to enter the mitochondrial matrix for β-oxidation, and ultimately ketone body synthesis.

COMPARISON OF FA OXIDATION AND FA SYNTHESIS

Table 5.3 and **Figure 5.8** show a couple of ways to compare and contrast the pathways of β-oxidation and fatty acid synthesis. **Table 5.3** summarizes key distinguishing features of the two pathways, such as cellular locations of the pathways, carriers of the intermediates, and forms of reducing power formed or used.

Table 5.3: Features distinguishing β-oxidation (FA oxidation) and FA synthesis

FEATURE	β-OXIDATION	FA SYNTHESIS
Location of pathway in cell	Mitochondria	Cytosol
Carrier of intermediate acyl groups	CoA-SH	ACP-SH
Organization of enzymes	None	FA Synthase Complex
Form in which 2-carbon units participate	Acetyl CoA	Malonyl CoA
Electron donor or acceptor used	FAD, NAD+	NADPH
Participation of CO_2	No	Yes
Stereochemistry of β-hydroxyacyl intermediate	L	D

Figure 5.8 compares the four repeated steps of β-oxidation of fatty acids with the four "key" repeated steps of fatty acid synthesis. On the right side of **Figure 5.8** is β-oxidation, while the left side shows fatty acid synthesis. The organization of the reactions is analogous to the oxidation states flow chart (**Figure 1.7**) in that the molecules become more oxidized as one moves "down" the page. As one moves "up" the page, the molecules are more reduced. The reactions on the right for β-oxidation go

"down" the page and are (1) dehydrogenation (a.k.a. oxidation), (2) hydration (3) dehydrogenation (a.k.a. oxidation), (4) thiolytic cleavage. On the left, start at the bottom and go "up" to carry out (1) condensation, (2) reduction, (3) dehydration (4) reduction. Also pay attention to whether the carrier is coenzyme A (β-oxidation) or the acyl carrier protein (ACP) for fatty acid synthesis.

Figure 5.8: Comparison of the four repeated steps of FA oxidation and FA synthesis pathways

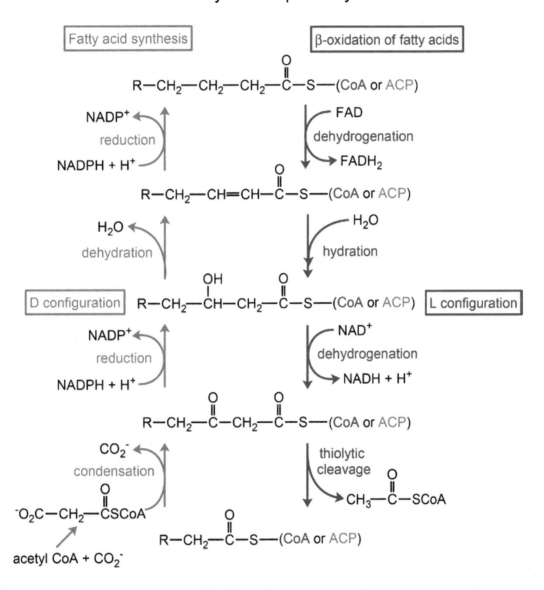

CPSIA information can be obtained
at www.ICGtesting.com
Printed in the USA
LVOW05s2040190816

501104LV00004BA/8/P

9 781621 312499